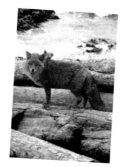

Nancy Sydnam

Sideways
Rain

. .

Hardscratch Press ❧ 2012

Sideways
Rain

*20 years of medicine, music, and
good-luck landings in the Aleutian
and Pribilof Islands of Alaska*

by NANCY ELLIOTT SYDNAM, M.D.

The background photograph of Akutan Island on the front and back covers and the rainy-day window on the front cover are by Daryl Moistner (www.nevadasurveyor.com), a good friend to Hardscratch Press. The back-cover photos of Nancy Sydnam and Tigger at Adak and of Atka village are from the author's collection. Unless otherwise noted, all photographs within the book are also from Dr. Sydnam's collection.

The frontispiece photo and the article headlined "Girl Medical Student Wins In Chilliwack Ploughing Test" are from Page 1 of the *Vancouver Sun*, Vancouver, B.C., July 7, 1949.

Nancy Sydnam's poetry has appeared in several journals: "Washington's Birthday," *Ice-Floe: International Poetry of the Far North*, Vol. II, No. 1, Summer Solstice 2001; "Fox Highway," *Inside Passages*, 2002; "Artist in Waiting," *Inside Passages*, 2002; "Gift," *Explorations*, 2002; "Anticipation," *Ice-Floe*, Vol. VII, No. 1, Summer Solstice 2006.

Printed in the United States of America.

First printed December 2012.

HARDSCRATCH PRESS, 658 Francisco Court, Walnut Creek, California 94598-2231.

www.hardscratchpress.com

Library of Congress Control Number: 2012953967

ISBN: 978-0-9838628-2-6

Cataloging-In-Publication Data

Sydnam, Nancy Elliott.
    Sideways rain : 20 years of medicine, music, and good-luck landings in the Aleutian and Pribilof Islands of Alaska / Nancy Elliott Sydnam.
        p. ; cm.
Includes bibliographical references and index.
ISBN: 978-0-9838628-2-6

    1. Sydnam, Nancy Elliott. 2. Physicians – Alaska – Biography. 3. Medical care – Alaska – Aleutian Islands – History. 4. Medical care – Alaska – Pribilof Islands – History. 5. Aleutian Islands (Alaska) – History. 6. Pribilof Islands (Alaska) – History. I. Title.

R154.S93A3 2012

2012953967

2 4 6 8 9 7 5 3 1

*Dedicated to the people
of the islands.*

Foreword

NANCY SYDNAM'S REMARKABLE BOOK accomplishes an almost impossible task. It presents an uncompromisingly frank yet compassionate portrait of one of the most diverse and remote regions of Alaska. As a physician who served the communities of Atka, Adak, Nikolski, St. George, St. Paul, Unalaska and Dutch Harbor from 1988 to 2010, she gleaned intimate knowledge of individuals and communities. She never betrays this intimacy, but uses it to illumine the strengths and attitudes that she came to admire in Aleut people and in those who moved to the Aleutians and the Pribilofs to live and work.

There are surprises in every chapter, from the traumas and reckless courage that surface in fast-paced fishing towns to the calm and melancholy that shroud these isolated villages on occasion. We share the frustrations inherent in traveling throughout the Chain. A cello appears unexpectedly and, along with Sydnam's devoted black Lab, remains a key character in the story. Over the course of the book, we come to know the author as a remarkable woman, a dedicated physician, an Alaskan original.

Because medicine was what brought Sydnam to the Chain, medical experiences chart the direction of the book and define its parameters. No one conveys the realities of Bush medicine better: the wide range of needs, the varied and dedicated practitioners, the struggles with bureaucracy, and the terrifying results of reduced or delayed services. She does this with frankness, humor, exactitude, and grace.

This exquisite mosaic is a moving and accurate journey through Aleutian communities at the end of one century and the beginning of another.

—Raymond L. Hudson,
author of *Moments Rightly Placed: An Aleutian Memoir*
and *Family After All: Alaska's Jesse Lee Home*
(Vol. I, Unalaska, 1889-1925)

Girl Medical Student Wins
In Chilliwack Ploughing Test

CHILLIWACK, April 7. — A girl pre-medical student at University of Washington in Seattle went back to the land Wednesday and won first prize in the novice class of the twenty-seventh annual ploughing match of the Chilliwack Ploughing Society.

Miss Nancy Elliott of Lynden, Wash., only woman competitor in the horse-drawn ploughing contests showed a pretty pair of heels to G. Jones, her male competitor, to win the Horatio Webb Trophy.

More than 2000 spectators watched Arthur Pahl, RR1, Chilliwack, become champion ploughman by piling up the largest number of points gained by any entrant in the 13 contests fought on the fields of Thompson Brothers' farm on Young Road.

The show, opened by Agriculture Minister Frank Putnam, also featured an impressive display of 65 of the latest farm implements and tractors. These, with teams and tractors entered in the match, took part in a parade through Chilliwack which preceded the match.

Champion Pahl succeeds William Shepherd of Steveston, the 1948 champ, who did not enter the competition this year.
Oldest pl----

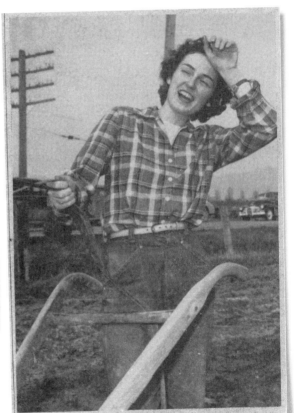

ONLY PLOUGHGIRL in the contest, pretty 20-year-old Nancy Elliott, of Lynden, Wash., handsomely won her trophy in the novice class. She defeated Glenn Jones of Chilliwack to capture the Horatio Webb trophy.

Table of Contents

*Note: Some journal entries cover a span of weeks;
the entries here give the opening date.*

. .

A Roundabout Route
to the Aleutians

"A Yukon Clinic"

In thirty providentially sunny days from 3 June through
3 July, 1961, my wife, a nurse, and Mr. John Spahn, a Guild
Optician, and I held an itinerant eye, nose and throat
and dental clinic in the Yukon Valley of Alaska. We were
accompanied on this safari by Nancy Sydnam, a general
practitioner of Anchorage. Dr. Sydnam went under the aegis
of the Alaska chapter of the American Cancer Society and
will report upon her observations in a separate communication. The remaining expenses were underwritten for the
most part by the other three members of the group.
The clinic was conducted, as the bureaucrats have it,
"at no expense to the government. . . ."

—Milo H. Fritz, M.D.,
Northwest Medicine, *Vol. 60, December 1961.*

MY LOVE AFFAIR WITH THE ALASKAN BUSH BEGAN in 1961 when I was privileged to participate as a general practice physician in a monthlong medical safari with Milo Fritz, a marvelous eye, ear, nose and throat physician (EENT). The trip to remote villages was initiated because Milo was concerned about ear infections and the resultant hearing problems so prevalent in the Bush. He had suggested to the Native Health Service that it do tonsillectomies and adenoidectomies (T&A's) on all problem cases. When the Native Service said it didn't have enough money to bring the estimated 250 cases to town, Milo said he would do the surgery in the villages. Following the example of the doctors aboard the cutter *Hygiene* years before, he would be doing surgery in a group of Native villages with no electricity other than an occasional generator, no plumbing, no hospital. Our hosts dipped water for surgery from lakes or the river and carried it in buckets on a yoke to the place being used for surgery, where we boiled it on an outdoor Yukon stove to sterilize the necessary instruments.

Milo felt strongly that the government agencies worked far too hard on doing things "for" or "to" the Native people and not nearly enough "with" them. As he explained in an article he wrote for *Northwest Medicine* in 1961:

> The clinic motto was, "Education, Participation, and Responsibility." We permitted any interested villager to watch everything we did from dental extractions and refractions to ether

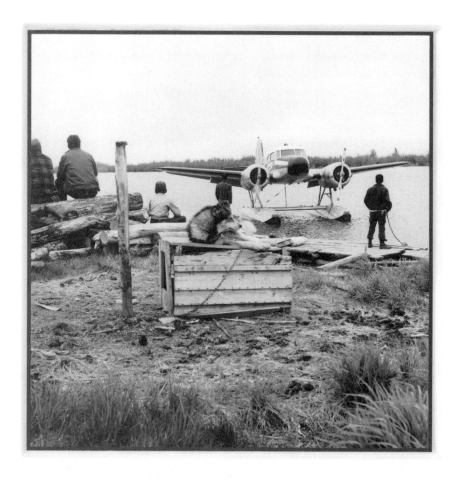

THEN AS NOW, *the rivers were the roads as well as the "runways" linking Bush communities with the rest of the world.*

anesthesia and T&A cases and tonsillectomies done under local anesthesia. This was the education.

In each village from eager volunteers we chose one girl to be my surgical assistant, one to scrub instruments, one to change scrub basins and keep alcohol rinse basins full, one to sit with the post operative patients and six boys to be ambulance crew. This constituted participation. None of these eager volunteers had passed the sixth grade in formal education, but all made up by eagerness, willingness, and heroic ability their formal education deficiencies.

In each village we had a collapsible army cot supplied by a Native family and this was used as the ambulance to carry the post-operative patients back to their cabins after recovery from the anesthesia. Supplying the cot was the responsibility of the ambulance crew along with promptness in appearing for duty. The responsibility of each parent or foster parent was for the appearance of his children at the proper time with a blanket and without having anything by mouth after midnight of the evening before or after breakfast at eight o'clock, if the child was scheduled for operation in the afternoon. We used our four air mattresses on the floor for the patients; the ambulance cot was bed number five.

Milo wanted and got the complete cooperation of every village we visited, and in each one we were working *with* the people and not *for* them.

The chosen villages were Shageluk and Holikachuk on the Innoko River, Huslia and Allakaket on the Koyukuk, Stevens Village and Beaver on the Yukon, and Venetie above the Arctic Circle on the Chandalar. Each had populations of between 100 and 150. Milo was the leader of our group; John Spahn, an optometrist, prescribed glasses and regulated the ether machine after Milo had anesthetized the patient. Milo flew the two of them to the villages in his Piper Tri-Pacer on floats. Milo's wife, Betsy, a nurse, taught the girls how to be scrub-nurses. I did all the pre-op physicals and monitored the difficult patients—those with coexisting medical problems—during

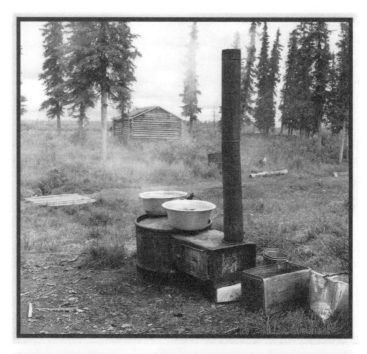

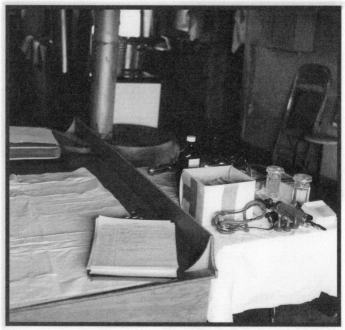

surgery. Betsy and I flew out commercially. There are no roads to these places—the river is the road. In the Bush, IFR ("Instrument Flight Rules") stands for "I Follow the River" when the weather gets bad for flying.

Because most women in these rural areas had never had Pap smears, the American Cancer Society sponsored me to do breast and pelvic exams with Pap smears on as many village women as possible. This presented its own challenges. For one thing, there are no exam tables in the Bush. I once had to resort to using the bishop's desk. (Each Episcopal village has a special chair or desk for the bishop to use when he visits. Customarily it is for his use only, though he is there for only a few days at a time. Knowing Bishop Gordon, I was sure he wouldn't mind, but I must admit to never telling him.) With doing the exams on the women and keeping track of all Milo's surgical patients, I was plenty busy. Betsy was determined that we all look professional and let me know not to plan on wearing jeans like everyone in the village, but to wear skirts and long cotton stockings. I still have the pairs I bought for the visits. They are beige, with seams.

Our first stop on that trip was in Shageluk, and I often think of what a superior introduction to Bush life this was for me. We were greeted by Jean Dementi, a former Los Angeles public health nurse who had worked in the hospital in Fort Yukon, then in various villages down river along the Yukon. She had met her future husband, Jim, in Shageluk, married him, and now had a daughter the same age as mine. She was not only extremely capable but brilliant as well. In later years she was first ordained as a deacon in the Episcopal Church and then ordained as a priest. At our first dinner the repartee between Milo and Jean was delightful. Jean told of

Previous page: OUTDOORS AND IN, *with the villagers' help (and the bishop's desk) we managed quite well.*

being asked to go on the "What's My Line" television show. The interrogator, a bit patronizing, asked how she came to be married to a Native. She answered thoughtfully, "Propinquity, I guess." I think he was afraid to ask many more questions.

Jean said she had always wanted to write a book titled "A Broad Along the Yukon." One of the stories would be of attending a woman in labor in a log cabin on a below-zero day. These cabins are kept very warm in winter, and as the labor went on for some hours Jean got warm and sweaty. After many cups of tea, she also had a full bladder and made her way outside to the privy. The expectant mother labored on and Jean did not reappear. The family eventually became worried—the patient was nearing delivery and still Jean had not come back. They went out to check and Jean was delighted to see them. She was a large woman, and her sweat had frozen her firmly to the outhouse seat. Using warm water they managed to defrost her from the seat in time for the birth. A two "delivery" day.

The banter ended with Jean reading from the *Herter Bull of the Woods Cookbook*. Herter was then a leading outdoor equipment store. I still have and use our over-55-year-old Herter canoe. She read a spinach recipe that began creatively, "As everyone knows, spinach was the Virgin Mary's favorite food." We all dissolved in laughter and got ready for the upcoming work.

And work we did. Jean had everything well organized, and the villagers enthusiastically pitched in. As planned, the girls were the scrub nurses, the boys the stretcher bearers, and the grandmothers looked after patients in the recovery room. It warms the heart to observe a whole community co-operating to achieve a goal with no money being involved. I felt privileged to be involved in such a venture.

Some patients came from Holikachuk farther up the Innoko River. I especially remember one couple who arrived by houseboat.

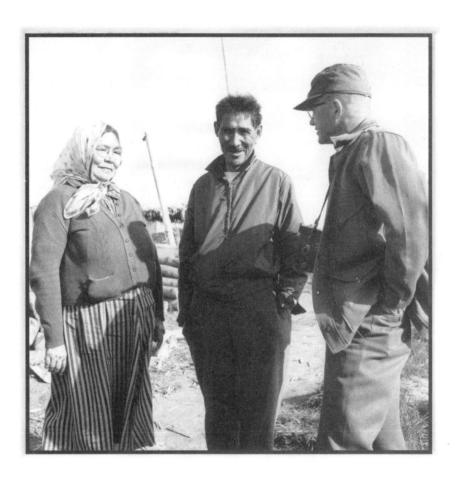

HOUSEBOAT OWNERS *from Holikachuk with* MILO FRITZ *(right).*

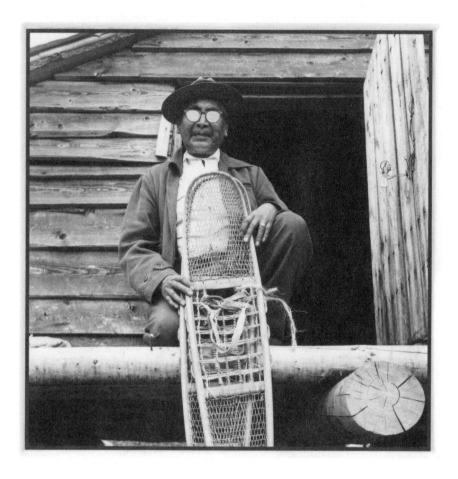

FUR TRAPPER *and snowshoe craftsman at Huslia.*

It was immaculately maintained, but best of all was the red fox bedspread on the double bed. The skins were beautifully matched and sewn—what artistry!

· ·

PART OF MY JOB WAS KEEPING a photographic record of the trip. I often took pictures of the interior of the village church because that is where I usually found the most beautiful decorative work in beads, skins and wood. The pure white moose-hide altar cloths were unbelievable.

The villagers were very generous with all of us, wanting us to enjoy their surroundings as much as they did. During "time-off" in Stevens Village I was loaned a canvas-covered kayak and went paddling on the Yukon. The quiet and the warmth of the sun were blissful. And I didn't have to wear the cotton stockings! The mosquitoes were not out yet, so after paddling some distance away from the village I relaxed and shed shirt and bra, reveling in the solitude and sun.

In Stevens Village I discovered a bad heart murmur in a young girl. Bishop Gordon had flown into town to see how we were doing—he always flew his own plane, a single-engine Cessna 180 called the "Blue Box" because it was purchased with the donations in the blue box most Episcopalians keep and use. He agreed to fly the girl in to Fairbanks for evaluation. As always, he cared for his flock.

In the village of Beaver I was able to deliver a woman of a healthy baby girl. What pleasure there is in safely delivering a woman of her baby in a log cabin! It is very different from working in a hospital where one has the latest technology, not to mention blood on hand if needed.

Huslia was unique among the villages because it had a community well. Instead of water being hauled from lakes or streams it was available from a pump right in the village. What a difference that made for easing some of the work of everyday life. Here I met another interesting elder, a trapper who was nearly blind because of cataracts. The kind owners of sled dogs let him use their dogs. He would set out with the dogsled, and the dogs knew where to stop to check traps. He would feel his way to the traps and use that same sense to retrieve any animal in the trap, while the dogs waited patiently for him. Then on they would go to the next one. As an experienced trapper he was able to finish the job if one of the animals was not yet dead. He also built and sold snowshoes, which he stained with some red substance from the ground. He grooved the wood so he could feel where to make attachments. I bought a pair of child's snowshoes for my son Elliott, who was two at the time, and they are still in very good condition.

· ·

THE INDIAN VILLAGE OF ALLAKAKET was just across the river from Alatna, an Eskimo village. These two communities demonstrated the long history of Eskimo/Indian conflicts in cultural border zones. It was obvious that little sharing went on between the two. I did enjoy meeting the priest in Allakaket. He had a window installed in the outhouse door so that one could look out at the beauty of the forest and hills instead of studying the ubiquitous Sears catalog. He also had marvelous recordings of classical music that he played in the evening while sipping a genteel glass of brandy.

In our time-off in Allakaket we were invited to a game of volleyball. Of course we joined in, not noticing how well-worn the area around the net was. We added to village pride by being skunked soundly. What a group of athletes! Now we understood why the area was so well worn—these folks played often and hard.

The last village we visited was Venetie, above the Arctic Circle. By then I could understand fully why Jean Dementi would spend her life happily working along the Yukon. In Venetie I was privileged to talk with one of the elders who had been on the original migration from the coast of the Beaufort Sea, on the Arctic Ocean, across the mountains of the Brooks Range. This was no stroll through the woods—the Brooks Range has peaks between eight and nine thousand feet. I visited her in her tent set up next to her daughter's house. When I entered I was amazed to see the floor covered by a woven willow rug much like the Japanese tatami. It was the most orderly tent I have ever seen. The woman had great presence. It filled the tent. She told me of the migration and how difficult it was. They had set off from the coast looking for a site with a more abundant food supply. Starving and exhausted from the long trip through the mountains, they could go no farther so camped and sent some of the strongest of the group ahead to see if there was any chance of finding food for survival. In a few days the scouts returned with caribou meat and a feast was held amidst much rejoicing. They were able to continue their journey to this land of plenty.

I too got to enjoy this land of plenty. I had never caught a grayling on a fly so I borrowed some gear and set off for the river. What a thrill to see that big dorsal fin leap out of the water. And the fish was delicious as well!

At the end of the trip all four of us were filled with good feelings. One was satisfaction for doing a much-needed job well. Milo performed more than 125 T&A's, most using ether anesthesia and a few under local. He had not a single complication. I, too, felt satisfaction, having assisted him with pre-ops as well as doing exams and Pap smears on the village women.

Another feeling was gratitude for the opportunity to spend an entire month with people who related so well to living on this earth as a part of this earth, rather than as masters of it. No wonder I refer to this as my love affair with the Alaskan Bush.

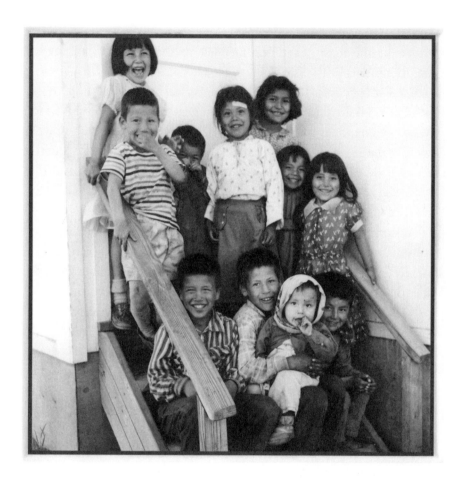

The playful children *at Stevens Village in 1961
are probably grandparents now.*

. .

My love affair with the Aleutian Islands began years later, in 1988, when I began thinking of divorcing myself from my 35-year marriage to a busy private practice as a family physician in Anchorage. I loved my practice and enjoyed giving cradle-to-grave care to three generations of families, but I had become disenchanted by the changes in medicine made by third-party payment. How could someone in an insurance office who had no medical education and who could not see the patient tell me what tests to order, or how long my patient could stay in the hospital? I was also annoyed by the insistent demand of medical malpractice insurance companies to practice defensive medicine. Such a practice, I thought, made medicine seem a business of cookbook recipes instead of the kind I preferred—actually relating to my patients. I still loved medicine, but it was time for a change.

Don Hudson, an emergency room doctor in the hospital where my office was located, was in charge of supplying physicians on a rotating basis to supervise three physician's assistants (PA's) staffing the Iliuliuk Clinic on Unalaska Island, 792 air miles southwest of Anchorage. There were no permanent physicians on any of the Aleutian Islands. News of unrest travels fast in the medical community, and Don asked if I might be available for intermittent encounters in the far-off and out-of-the-way Aleutians. He said he would keep in touch and hoped that I could decide within a week or so.

I thought about it. I would have to be gone from home for one or two weeks at a time, and the type of medicine would be vastly different from the staid family practice in which I knew all my patients. It could be difficult to be so far removed from any second opinion when needed and from the technology available in Anchorage. Yet it didn't sound too remote when I recalled with fondness the delightful monthlong safari along the Yukon in 1961. For that trip I had sent my then-4-year-old daughter, Claire, and son Elliott, age 2, to stay with my parents on their farm in Lynden, Washington, while I was away. They had a great time. (Elliott collected eggs with my father. Once while my father was hanging up his coat, Elliott put the eggs in a safe place where they wouldn't get broken—in the boots my dad had just removed. They were not found until the following morning. The results were quite a surprise but quickly forgiven.) My sons Bruce and Ben, born later in the '60s, missed this childhood adventure.

But these new trips I was considering would never last as long as a month, and because my children were grown and gone from home, I wouldn't have to be concerned about their care.

So—should I go to Unalaska? I knew nothing other than that it was a fishing port out on the chain. However, my interest was sparked by a recent trip to the Anchorage Museum. I had bought a beautiful soapstone and ivory sculpture of an Aleut woman sewing a *chixdax* (a gut or fish-skin raincoat). I had met the Aleut artist, Gert Svarny, and in conversation watched her face fill with delight as she spoke of the beauty of the mountains and the joy of eating fresh clams from the beach just yards in front of her home. She had invited me to her studio if I ever got to Unalaska. The stars seemed aligned, the balance tipping.

Supervise three PA's? I had enjoyed teaching Washington, Alaska, Montana, and Idaho (WAMI) medical students in my practice and knew I could teach PA's a thing or two. My teaching experience upped the degree of interest for both Don and me.

Don called again and waxed more eloquent. He described Unalaska as a small village on the northern end of Unalaska Island, and Dutch Harbor on adjacent Amaknak Island as accessible via "The Bridge to the Other Side." Dutch Harbor is the largest fishing port in the United States, he said—home to the fishing fleet of the Bering Sea and the North Pacific. The fishing industry would provide a large proportion of patients seen at the clinic; the rest would come from the village. As Don wooed me he told me how "varied and interesting" the practice was, and, "Oh, yes, the weather is interesting, too."

. .

As I WRESTLED WITH WHETHER to accept such a challenging change, I began to hear the same voices I had heard in my youth when all the boys (but none of the girls) got to go north to Alaska to fish every summer. Before the medical safari with Milo Fritz I had clearly heard my paternal grandfather whisper from his wagon on the Mullen Trail, as he headed west from Montana to Walla Walla, Washington, "You can do it. Just figure out how." I also recalled how my maternal great-aunt, Sarah, had run away from Scotland to America with her Irish sea-captain, taking only the hand-made linen sheets from home. (Years later, her granddaughter, my Aunt Joy, embroidered separate messages on a portion of those precious sheets when my sisters and I were born. Mine reads "Those in January born/can never be forlorn.") I had listened to these same voices when I decided to go to medical school and again when I arrived in Anchorage, Alaska, just out of internship in 1955. I was ready to listen to them again.

When I first started practice in Anchorage I was one of 16 physicians in a city of about 30,000. I soon got to know all the other doctors as well as who was good at what, so referrals turned out well. My husband and I lived in a little house on Sand Lake south of the airport, eight miles out in the country. The house had been built by an energetic pilot for Pacific Northern Airlines, for which my husband also worked as a dispatcher.

Because I had always idolized Amelia Earhart, I enjoyed the contact with all the pilots. One of them, Joe Stevens, taught me to fly in his Super Cub and I loved it. Baby number three, Robert Bruce, arrived in 1963; between pregnancies I eventually got my land and sea rating. (I found I could not get the stick back far enough to land when my pregnant uterus got in the way.) Flying really opened the country to me because there were so few roads; Anchorage had only three paved streets. I knew I had moved into the small-town practice I had wanted.

. .

IN THE LATE '50S PACIFIC NORTHERN was sold to Western Airlines, which wanted my husband to transfer to California. Leaving Alaska was unthinkable for both of us so Syd quit Pacific Northern and went to work for the state troopers as a dispatcher.

He advanced to trooper and worked his way up to Deputy Commissioner of Public Safety. My enjoyable Anchorage practice was interrupted when he was transferred to Juneau in 1967. We moved there with the three children and I worked part-time for two family practitioners as well as covering for the internist or the pediatrician when they needed vacations. I still refer to this time as my "five-year retreat."

I had a black lab named Max and a nice Ithaca 12-gauge pump shotgun. I would get the children off to school in the morning and then go duck hunting on the wetlands and lakes available in several directions less than three miles from home. One morning I was out with Max near the airport when I noticed a group of several men downing ducks but unable to retrieve them from the water. I was 39 years old and about seven months pregnant with Ben but waddled over to them to see if they would like the services of Max. They were astronauts on their way to "moon training" in the Valley of 10,000 Smokes on the Alaska Peninsula, where Katmai had erupted violently in 1912 leaving thousands of acres of utter desolation. Their hosts had offered duck hunting but had no dog. Max shone, retrieving a dozen ducks, one after another. The astronauts were impressed and I was proud of my Max.

Juneau offered mountains to climb and glaciers to explore plus wonderful bays and inlets safe for small boats. Coming from king crab heaven in Anchorage, I had always disdained the scrawny

Dungeness. Was I ever in for a lesson! Sunken crab pots are necessary to get crab, right? Wrong! In Juneau, with friends like Ron and Lois Naab, it was possible to chase the crustaceans with a boat and just dip them up in a landing net, thence to the pot of sea water boiling over the fire on the beach, and forget king crab. The Naabs' children were about the same ages as ours, and Lois and I had many wonderful adventures herding our children over beaches and across glaciers. The older ones kept the little ones in line by yelling, "If you don't keep up, the eagles will get you!"

Another of my Juneau friends, Diane Tickell, had decided to go to seminary and would be gone for a few years. She had a 14½-foot lap-strake Metlakatla dory and agreed to sell it to us for $100 if she could buy it back for the same amount when she returned. What a deal! A work-boat for Fish and Game, it was entirely seaworthy and safe for hauling kids around. Syd bent willows over the prow and attached a tarp so the children could stay dry. With a 10-horse outboard motor it gave us excellent access to all the coves and bays that called. One especially memorable day we anchored off an island outside of Auke Bay to fish. We were dozing in the sun and occasionally bobbing the bait when we heard a whooshing sound and immediately smelled something very fishy. A whale had just spouted next to the boat before diving. It was actually very gentle, and the boat barely rocked.

· ·

THE IDYLL ENDED IN 1972 when my husband was transferred back to Anchorage. In our absence oil had been discovered on the North Slope and the ambience of the community had changed drastically.

In the next 10 to 15 years Anchorage became a boom town, with hundreds of doctors and three newly built or enlarged hospitals, including a Native hospital, plus a military hospital on nearby Fort Richardson. The city justly became known as "Los Anchorage," because of its traffic problems. Our little Sand Lake, which had

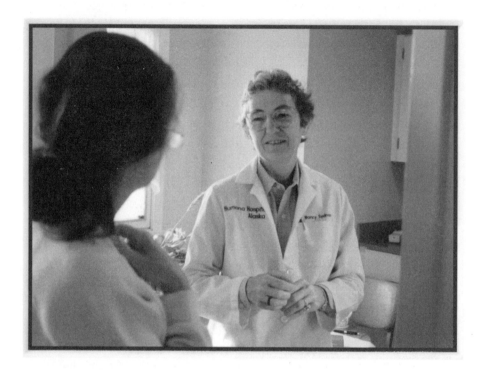

CALL IT OLD-FASHIONED, *but on all my*
assignments I "dressed" for work.

three houses on it when we moved there, suddenly had houses every 70–100 feet, with boats, water skiers and planes instead of swimming moose and shy lynx on the shore. Even the muskrat had moved from under our dock. That wasn't the only thing that had changed, however. Our 22-year marriage was insolvent. We divorced. I moved with the children downtown to a quiet neighborhood where the moose agreed to sleep under our mountain ash. It was close to the hospitals where I worked—Humana and Providence—for my expanding practice. I now shared office space with an obstetrician/gynecologist, Dr. Claire Renn, and we were both busy. In the ensuing years I hired first one and then a second family practitioner to help carry the family practice portion. While I still loved caring for my families, the changes occurring in medicine over those 16 years eroded the charm. Thus, when Don approached me, Unalaska and "Dutch" sounded more and more appealing.

．．

I HADN'T CLOSED MY PRACTICE. I now had two associates to share the load. What did I have to lose? I could have my cake and eat it too. I was only 60 and ready for a fling, and my grandfather and my Great-Aunt Sarah urged me on. I said, "Yes." Every two months I began taking a week from my insurance-directed practice, packing a few clothes, a stethoscope, some books, groceries and often a cello, to board a Reeve Aleutian Airways plane and head for a new experience. I hoped this adventure would bring the same satisfaction as the early years of my practice.

On my first trip out I took a large bag of oranges as a treat for the villagers. It was winter—cold and windy—and as I descended from the plane's last step the bag broke and I chased oranges rolling in the wind over the tarmac. What an entrance!

I was greeted by one of the PA's and taken to "quarters" (old World War II duplexes) on Standard Oil Hill near the airport on Amaknak Island. It snowed during the night. In the morning, with the PA driving, we passed streets named Bjorka, Kashega, Kovrizhka and Makushin as we plowed through drifts to work. We passed Bunker Hill on the right just before The Bridge to the Other Side, and, now on Unalaska Island, we skirted Haystack on our left and then crossed Iliuliuk Creek. A right turn led to the one-story clinic opposite the high school.

In the Unangan language Iliuliuk means "harmony" or "gathering of the people," and the clinic was certainly that. It was a busy place, doing its best to please. The ceiling leaked, the floor slanted. We had an x-ray machine that we used on our own. No lab techs, but we could do our own minor studies (hemoglobins, hematocrits, complete blood counts, differentials, urines). All other lab work was sent to Anchorage to be returned in a week or two, depending on weather. We had IV fluids available, but no blood. We had indoor plumbing and electricity, but there was no surgeon, no orthopedist, no hospital—we were it. One doctor and two or three PA's to take care of whatever arrived at our door. Phone numbers of various medical evacuation (medivac) teams we frequently used were prominently displayed. The teams came "weather permitting." Two Anchorage hospitals had medivac crews that rotated on-call times. The planes were equipped to handle medical emergencies. There were a couple of other companies as well as the ever-available Coast Guard and our local pilot, Tom Madsen, who did medivac flights in his Beechcraft or the amphibious Grumman Goose that he owned or perhaps leased.

The staff at the clinic was outstanding—careful, knowledgeable, and certainly kind to newcomers like me. Marlaine, my nurse, was excellent. She was from Texas, had a drawl, and never got flustered regardless of the medical dangers that frequently presented themselves.

The clinic did care for the village residents, but its main patient load came from the fishing industry. Several processors along shore in the bay served both the fishing and the crabbing boats. The accident rate was extremely high.

I was to learn what a sheltered life I had led in my family practice. Dutch Harbor attracted workers from all over the globe, including Russia, Scandinavia, South America, Somalia—anywhere there was a dearth of jobs. Unfortunately, sexually transmitted diseases followed, and I got a better lesson in that subject than even the big-city Philadelphia General Hospital, where I trained, could give me.

After my first trip to Dutch, the job and I seemed more compatible with each visit. When the clinic staff discovered how much experience I had in obstetrics, they wanted to hire me more often to help solve some of the problems faced by local pregnant women. The cost of flying to Anchorage from Unalaska/Dutch Harbor was close to a thousand dollars round trip, which made it unlikely that expectant mothers would make multiple trips to ensure a good outcome. As a result, they would arrive in Anchorage at a time near their due date without any of the preliminary lab work or necessary follow-up done. The clinic offered me a new job. They wanted me coming for two weeks every two months to develop an obstetrical protocol that would be comparable to what existed in Anchorage. At that point they planned to send Marlaine out for further training so that she could continue the care on an everyday basis. The goal, the job, the location suited me very well so I completed the divorce from my practice by selling it to my two associates in 1989. I went to work solely for the Iliuliuk Clinic. I was in for a wild ride.

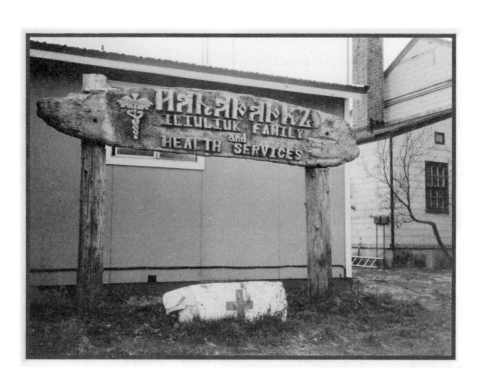

PART I

. .

The Iliuliuk Clinic

Airport ⫣ɑ·−⊏

I love this sideways Aleutian rain.
Instead of upright, it comes down prone.
(Dear God, please don't delay my plane.)

When I'm out here upon the Chain
I hear the Natives all intone,
"I love this sideways Aleutian rain."

Tourists tend to feel the strain.
Beneath their breath I hear them moan,
"Dear God, please don't delay my plane."

The hardy ones sing this refrain,
With coats around their shoulders thrown:
"I love this sideways Aleutian rain."

If there were tracks, I'd take the train,
For they'd be sure to get me home.
(Dear God, please don't delay my plane.)

I'm outward bound, I can't complain.
At least, it's all confirmed by phone.
I love this sideways Aleutian rain.
(Dear God, please don't delay my plane.)

THE MORE OFTEN I FLEW THE 800 MILES OUT TO MY new "office," the more respect I had for Reeve Aleutian Airways. It was founded in 1932 by Bob Reeve, who said, "I had to fly to eat and I'd finally found out how I could eat regular—by doing the kind of flying that no one else wanted." I always felt safe in a Reeve plane, even the one that had a sign over the exit that read "Escape Rope." The pilots seemed to have excellent judgment, knowing when to fly and when to turn around.

Almost all of my journal entries mention weather because it was a major factor in getting out there or getting home. Winds frequently gusted to 90 miles per hour, blowing down antennas and causing loss of communication between the island and the mainland where all our support lay. The World War II-era runway—there is only one—is closely adjacent to Mt. Ballyhoo, with the result that winds on opposite ends of the runway are often from opposite directions. In addition, the runway is fairly short, only 4,000 feet, and the ends frequently surrender to the sea during violent storms, which of course shortens it even more. The trick was to land as close to the near end of the runway as possible without catching the landing gear on the edge of the cliff on approach. Then immediately after the wheels touched down the brakes had to go on or the tailwind on the opposite end would hit, and off the plane would go into the bay on that end. It was always exciting. One newcomer airline once dragged a wingtip on the strip during landing and crashed, breaking the engine off the wing.

Takeoffs were equally exciting but not so prolonged. The pilot could try a go-around on landing. But if the pilot erred on takeoff the plane was in the drink with no second chance.

The trip from Anchorage to Dutch is scheduled to take three hours. If weather defeats landing you have to fly back to Cold Bay, about an hour away, or all the way to Anchorage, and then try again the next day. Pilots often don't want to admit failure (this wasn't true of Reeve). On a flight I was on one day the pilot made three attempts to land at Dutch, each more perilous than the last. He announced over the intercom that he was sorry to say we were to return to Anchorage. As one, the entire group cheered and clapped.

Boarding a plane to the Aleutians is not like going to San Francisco or New York City. There are no cozy covered ramps. Passengers walk in any kind of weather out to the plane on the tarmac and then climb the steep stairs up into the fuselage. When I have fragile baggage—for instance, my cello—I carry it out to the plane and only then, before climbing the stairs, do I give it to the baggage handler to gently insert into the hold instead of relying on the old heave-ho.

Carting a cello around is a pain, especially in the Aleutians, and probably doesn't make sense to people who have never played a musical instrument. I played in the Anchorage Civic Orchestra before I began the itinerant life that made me miss too many rehearsals. There was such deep satisfaction in everything from practice to rehearsal to performance with the entire orchestra that I hated to give it up. I felt like a toreador when I donned my "concert black" before a performance, then stood when the conductor entered, and applauded him by patting my cello to produce a pleasant resonance. I can say all sorts of things musically that could never be communicated in words; in the orchestra there was also the joy of working very hard as a group to produce something memorable that might touch the innermost parts of our audience. My cello is my companion on the road as well as at home. When I travel with it I usually encounter other musicians who want to join in for our mutual enjoyment. One time I found a retired concert pianist out in Naknek on Bristol Bay, and did we ever have fun.

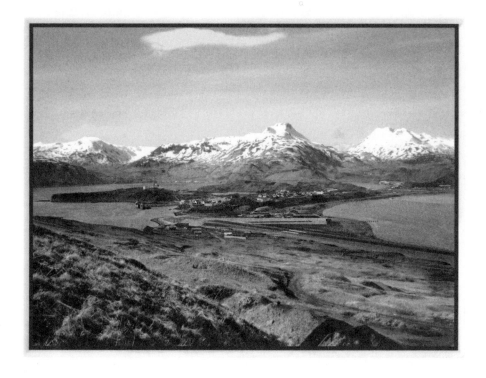

Unalaska/Dutch Harbor, *the infamous runway in the middle distance, extending from center to right side of photograph.*

Dutch Harbor

... *Feb. 19, 1991 — Tuesday.*

ANCHORAGE WEATHER WAS GOOD FOR TAKEOFF, but winds were high in Dutch. Nevertheless all passengers boarded at the scheduled time. Then we sat and sat. The planes we board have routinely been sitting out in the weather without their engines running, so there is no heat. I have learned to wear insulated boots on flights. After a very long wait, the airline announced the flight had been canceled. We all deplaned and I picked my cello up and hefted it back to baggage claim to get the rest of my luggage.

Before I could call a taxi and leave for home to try again the next day, they announced the weather was clearing and there would be a later flight. There was at least a chance it might get there so I rebooked, rechecked bags and once again trudged out to the plane with my cello. All of us were happy to have another chance to get there at least on the appointed day. We took off and made it past Cold Bay, the usual "turn-around" or "wait for weather" spot about two-thirds of the almost-800-mile flight to Dutch Harbor.

We continued on in gorgeous weather until descent and landing near Dutch Harbor, where we pitched about in heavy turbulence and then, low over the water, wheeled right over Iliuliuk Bay past the spit. At the last moment the pilot flattened the plane's 45-degree bank and plopped it on the end of the runway—a few bounces, full reverse thrust and we were there.

It was too late to go to work, so Pat, the clinic manager, took me straight to my Unisea duplex, the same one as the last visit. The weather was clear and cold with minor winds. All the mountains were lovely with new snow. A NW wind, so flocks of birds were on Margaret Bay just in front of the house. This time I had binoculars and a bird book. There was a huge flock of old squaw ducks and harlequins too, plus common goldeneyes—and today I saw some eiders. Nice to have the time to settle in. I put things away while I watched birds and then went to get groceries. The few blocks to the grocery store are always a nice walk.

I had soup for dinner and then practiced about half an hour on the cello after first closing the doors of both the bedrooms so I wouldn't disturb the neighbors, whom I've never heard. Mickey, Clare and I are trying to work something up for music at a church service. Today I gave the Hayden trio music to Clare, one of the best FNP's (family nurse practitioners). She plays the violin. I'll try to deliver the piano parts to Mickey, the school music teacher, tomorrow.

Sure nice to have my cello here to play. This is my student cello (I am the student, not the cello). I have now decided that rather than subject it to the perils of travel and delivery by forklift I will leave it at the clinic to play when I come. I will have to bring only my bow on the plane, while keeping my performance cello at home.

We had a beast of a day at the clinic. Lots of sick people and some good confirmations of diagnoses I'd made last time here. (Best was endometriosis, a diagnosis I made on the basis of history and physical without the benefit of ultrasound, which we don't have here.) I saw a patient for Rick, one of the

PA's. The patient was a 39-year-old man with sudden onset of abdominal pain this morning after a shower. No fever, but white blood cell count (WBC) of 17,000 and severe shortness of breath (orthopnea). I gave IV fluids and watched as his belly got hard. I thought it might be inflammation of the abdominal membranes (peritonitis) of some kind. He had a wet cough and his WBC—indication of infection—continued to rise while his measures of blood concentration (hemoglobin and hematocrit) fell. I couldn't believe blood loss, though; thought septic shock more likely. Medivac finally got here at 6 p.m. as I was leaving. His pulse was 100–112 (normal 60–80), BP 130/60 (from 60/30 initially). He wasn't pale anymore. My guess is hot appendix—maybe pneumonia with secondary peritonitis. Far out would be acute pancreatitis or leaking aortic aneurysm. His upright x-ray showed no air under the diaphragm so he didn't perforate a gut. Chest film was worthless. Still had high-pitched bowel sounds when I left. I am so glad he got out.

(Postscript [2-20-91]: He had a 3-day-old ruptured spleen! His belly was full of blood. Three days ago he was hit in the stomach, which must have partially ruptured his spleen, and the day before his symptoms began, he lifted 100# boxes all day, which exacerbated the problem. The surgeon in Anchorage made his incision for an appy and was probably as surprised as I was to find his belly full of blood, so at least I had company in thinking appendicitis. He was doing well the last I heard.)

As I walked home the streets seemed empty compared with last time I was here. I didn't see any boats tied up to the

Barge Inn either. It really is a barge, left over from the Prince William Sound spill clean-up when it was used for crew housing. Someone pulled it here and set it up as a floating hotel. Not bad since rooms are hard to find. Margaret Bay is only 15–20 feet in front of my duplex, which is the last one next to the storage yard. There is a skim of ice on the NW part tonight so the birds aren't as close as they were yesterday. No sea lions so far. I'll have to take my circular walk past A/C (Alaska/Commercial, general store) and around to the western beach tomorrow. I am too tired tonight. The sea lions like it near western beach because when the canneries flush their liquid fish waste it floats out of the inner harbor and ends up near the beach over there. I saw 6–8 sea lions last time I was here. They are so funny with their acrobatic antics. I can never tell quite what part I am seeing with all the leaps and body parts flying around. I hear they pull out on the little reef just to the right of my place sometimes. I'd love to be that close to them.

No newspaper tonight. They were all gone by the time I got to the store—of course. I sure have to laugh at one bundle of papers for 5,000 people. Timing is all. Last time I managed to get a Sunday paper, and that was a real coup!

2-20-91

WEDNESDAY—COLD, CLEAR and windless this morning. Unusual! Almost all my little bay is frozen over and even in this early light I can see Mt. Newhall outlined against the sky. It is going to be a beautiful day, and unlike yesterday there is both heat and hot water in the unit. I am basking in comfort.

2-23-91

SATURDAY—WE HAD A great and invigorating storm Friday with snow, wind, and finally, sleet. Jan drove me home and I loved seeing the steely blue-gray and green of the water with its flecks of foam. Boats were coming and going as though the storm were immaterial. I love the boat names—*Neptune, Lady Louise, Aurora, Kara Gail, Miss Leona, Boxer.* There are two more "dog boats"—the *Retriever* and the *Labrador*— but I have not seen them yet.

I had a hurried dinner and then went off up the valley to Rita's place for bridge. What a lovely home! Rita and her husband bought an old 16×20-foot WW II cabana and rebuilt it. Now it has a spacious living room, dining room and kitchen tastefully furnished and decorated. It even has hardwood floors. Typical Alaskan porch with a sign that reads "Please remove your shoes." Two tables set for bridge. The games were awful, with a lot of learners, but the company was excellent. Mary is a magistrate, Cat, a comptroller. Rita works for the city in some capacity, and Shelly teaches first grade. I can't really remember all the rest. AB Rankin, longtime city treasurer, was there and had made lemon meringue pie that was delicious! None of them drink, or at least, no alcohol was served. I scraped the sleet off Mary's car and went home about midnight.

The storm is over this morning, though I haven't heard any planes. High tide brings a constant parade of ducks past my door. The Steller's eider are spectacular with their gaudy patterns. I always thought eider were large birds but these are small—about the size of bufflehead. I had trouble eating breakfast with my eyes glued to the binoculars and the bird book. I could easily spend the day watching them, especially because they are so close.

Yesterday at noon, in a howling onshore gale, I walked over to Nicky's Place, the local, very good bookstore on the Unalaska side. When I came out, there was the *Mr. B* steaming into harbor—a squat, ugly white boat with a blue band around it. I wished I had a camera to take a picture of it for my son Ben, who worked aboard her one summer. But with the snow blowing so hard I could barely see it, so the photo probably wouldn't have made it. I saw it at anchor last night and was going to take a picture this morning but it was already gone. Ben probably doesn't really want a reminder of his scabies nest anyway. Hygiene on fishing boats is never very good. Long hours of work and I suspect no one ever changes bunk linen. Sometimes more than one hand shares a bunk, with one sleeping while the other works.

Mickey, the school music teacher, called yesterday, and our music group is to meet today at noon at the school. He rounded up a flute player so it should be fun. We were to meet at three but he called to say he had forgotten he was on a rope-jumping team at three. I think it's like "Walk for Hope" only they jump rope for the lung association. I love small towns. I had no idea how I missed them until I came here.

2-25-91

MONDAY—YESTERDAY I decided that I would just stay home and rest. It was a good decision. All the birds in the bay paraded past my window, plus a few seals and two kinds of eagles (the young birds don't look like adults, plus there are sometimes what I think are golden eagles around—very confusing), scaup, scoters, mergansers, goldeneyes, Steller's eiders, old squaw and harlequins. It was grand and I am getting better at identifying them—I think. At least the seals are a cinch.

I heard the jet land at about two or three and walked to the store for the Sunday paper. I was too early so walked along the dock. Boats were parked three deep and there was activity on all of them. Ice hung from lots of the rigging. I wish I had taken my camera. There is never a time when I can't hear some boat running, except when it gets drowned out by loud storms. I managed to get my paper and spent the remainder of a restful day at home.

The receptor dish was blown off-center in a recent storm and not recalibrated, so I no longer get radio reception. However, I do have nice music tapes that Harold Borofsky, the husband of Leatrice, one of my med school cadaver partners, made to play. But I miss "Radio Reader" on NPR at night. The reader was almost to the end of a good book.

2-26-91

TUESDAY—THIS EVENING, after a long and hard day's work, we did play music and it was great. Barbara Crandall on flute is excellent. Clare has been trained as a luthier, and her homemade violin has wonderful tone. We played for almost three hours. The pieces are varied and pleasant and, with a little work, well within our abilities. We set up a second practice for tomorrow night at seven. I will have to rush dinner a bit, but I'm looking forward to it. After practice tonight we stopped in at the clinic to pick up a radio (one of the small,

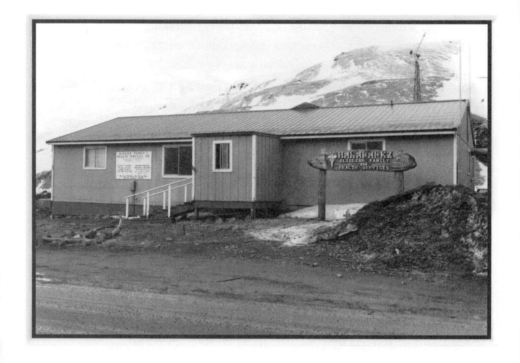

THE BELOVED *old Iliuliuk Clinic building.*

hand-held, two-way sets we use). The place was swamped with patients so I said I'd start dinner (to which I'd invited Clare), and then come back. We worked like dogs until 8:30. Did the stew ever smell good when I walked in! I called Clare to let her know I was home and she walked over. Another nice evening with good conversation.

Tonight it is rainy and windy—just right for sleeping. Sure glad I don't have to take night call.

2-27-91

WEDNESDAY—AT 6 A.M., when I get up, it is too dark to tell what kind of day it will be, but yesterday was strictly "Aleutian," with pelting rain and strong gusty winds, SE I think. No planes since Sunday. My bay is almost devoid of ducks. I rushed home from work at 5:30 p.m. to have dinner before our music practice at 7. Fortunately both halves of the duplex have great kitchens so cooking is easy, leaving time to stare out the window. The bay was that lovely gray-green with froth all over. Rain against the windows made for bad visibility but I happened to see a sea lion leap all the way out of the water. I swear he was playing in the rough water. I grabbed the binoculars and by standing on the davenport and looking out the very top of the window I was able to find an unobscured spot. He was wonderful! At first I could see his head, then he must have been foraging on the shallow bottom because just his flippers would be up, splashing about. Then he would tear around and jump out again. I was late to practice. It was better than Sea World! Practice was great fun. I didn't get home until 10 or so.

I had a patient from Israel yesterday. I wondered what he is doing over here, other than making money. He and I spoke briefly of the current war and agreed that it was nonsense with conflicts going back centuries. I saw Abi (not to be confused with AB), the owner of Nicky's Place, later and she knew all about this man. He had been living on a kibbutz when some sort of conflict began near the northern border. Members of his family had died in concentration camps, and the sounds of war and the ambulances freaked him out, so he decided to leave Israel and travel the world. She met him one day when he came into her office at the store. He was carrying a 30- or 50-gallon black plastic bag that held something "roundish" and heavy. It almost looked like the bag was full of water because even the square corners were full and poking out. He began talking excitedly, asking if she could tell him "what this is." She said she would try.

At this he put the bag down on her office rug where it squooshed out in a flattish shape. He spread newspapers from his day-pack on the floor, gently placed the bag on them, opened it and spread the sides out and down. It was a jellyfish about 30 inches in diameter! She was amazed to see it—a "lion's mane" jellyfish, one of the group that swarms and ranges all the way from California to Alaska. It kind of oozed out of the bag and onto the newspapers and was gorgeous. When it finally settled, Abi said, it was at least 5–7 inches thick. It had clear, still jelly around the outside ring, and the center was a ruffled mass with color from deep orange egg yolk to a kind of burnt orange. She had never seen one so intact and perfect and here was this three-foot-wide specimen on her office floor! She told me she talked with him for about an hour asking all kinds of questions interspersed with his questions to her. Who was he? Where did he find this? Where was he from? Was this creature heavy? Were there more? Do you think this is edible? Why was he there? How did he get it into the bag? Did he get stung?

What an education one can get in a bookstore next to the Bering Sea! I suppose I should give some idea of what Abi is like since it might explain why a Jewish immigrant would bring his prize catch to her for identification.

My first experience of Abi's unique talent occurred as we were driving the back road to Summer Bay. The light was just right, showing all the strata of the cliffs we passed as Abi described them in detail. (She had, after all, been there many times on her motorcycle looking for the right kind of lichen to dye yarn royal purple, and incidentally knew that the urine of very young boys was exactly the right ph to hold the color.) She told me that whenever she and her mother took trips, back in the '50s, Abi would take dictation from her mother for her book, *Roadside Geology of Connecticut*. Abi's mother was the director of the Children's Museum of Hartford, which meant that Abi grew up in the museum world of the East Coast, getting a wonderful foundation in geology, botany, marine biology, history and art. With her innate intelligence and unending curiosity she acquired a tremendous breadth of knowledge that did not go unnoticed in Unalaska.

I am always interested in who from the parochial East Coast manages to arrive in the Aleutian Islands. Abi had always wanted to study sub-arctic anthropology, so she transferred to the University of Alaska Fairbanks. After about nine years there she moved with her husband to Kodiak. In 1974, when her husband was fishing "out west" in the Bering Sea, Abi decided to leave Kodiak and go west as well. She hitched a ride on a crab boat headed to Unalaska and encountered a vicious storm on the way. Was she sick and frightened down below? No, she was in the pilot house learning to calculate the height of the waves (50 ft.!) by triangulation. Another Aleutian Islander was born. In 1980 Abi and her business partner, Kathy Grimnes, started the bookstore, which Abi ran after Kathy went to work running the local Native corporation. Nicky's Place is across the street from the Elbow Room, Unalaska's rowdy bar. She occasionally has to clean the store's porch of the blood left over from fights the previous night.

2-28-91

THURSDAY—THAT WIND I spoke of a day or so ago was up to 80 knots, and some ships began dragging anchor, so rather than let them blow ashore or into each other, the harbormaster made them put to sea. I wondered why there were so many off Mt. Ballyhoo (the 1,634 ft. mountain next to the runway on Amaknak Island) when I went to work yesterday morning.

Unalaska

April 16, 1991 — Tuesday.

THE FLIGHT TO UNALASKA WAS EASY THIS TIME. I am housed in a lovely new townhouse only a block from the clinic. I miss my view of the water and all its activity but I will probably practice cello more this time. I will get used to Carl's grocery here instead of A/C, which is over on Amaknak Island. Again, all are within walking distance. I am one minute from Town Creek and two minutes from the beach on Iliuliuk Bay where Gert Svarny used to dig clams. My kind of town.

4-24-91

WEDNESDAY—WHAT A difference locale makes! With no bay as a background, I just haven't done any writing. Unalaska is certainly much more quiet than Dutch. It is rather like a residential area as compared with business. Here Dutch is referred to as "the other side" and one doesn't take one's children there since it is so blatantly drug-oriented, with dealing and usage openly taking place all over. State troopers can't help because it is city jurisdiction.

I did get out to "glass beach" on Sunday (so called because that is where the military dump was). A fair day so I walked over. I saw a ground squirrel that was quite tame. There were many harlequin ducks but the eider had gone. One lone sea lion. I walked my old loop past the duplex, got a Sunday paper at A/C and took a cab home (point A to point B for $5).

When Erin, the fill-in PA, left I got use of the clinic car and drove to the antenna on Ballyhoo, the other side of the airport. I climbed down a very steep cliff to Fossil Beach. I love the surf and the sand and even though I didn't find any fossils, I did see a sea otter fairly close. I went back up my cliff, hand over hand, and chased a few eagles trying to get a better look. Saw two of what I thought were goldens but were probably just juveniles, and two beautiful balds on the cliff near the beach. Two of those enormous sea eagles flew off before I could dig my binoculars out of my bag. Abi says the big ones are probably juveniles. Because they don't know how to fly very well they have longer feathers to compensate, and that makes them look larger than the adults.

It looks to be a good day today. It sure isn't as stormy as in winter. I expect an easy trip home.

Activity has been very slow at the clinic since the bottom fishery season for pollock closed. I am sure things will be hopping again in short order. It is nice to have a lull and not be completely exhausted at night. I had a 31-year-old man with pus in his chest (empyema). His pulse was 140 and respirations 40. He certainly was sick. I put a chest tube in and sent him to Anchorage. I think he made it. The report said it was pneumococcal.

· ·

May 29, 1991 — Wednesday

I'M IN THE SECOND WEEK OF A FANTASTIC STAY. I was too busy to write during the first week. My sister Ann came out with me and had a wonderful time. She is a couple of years younger than I am. Her husband of over 40 years died last year, and rather than have her sit at home bereft I now invite her to come out and see something new. One of her daughters works for Alaska Airlines so travel is no problem for her. While I worked, she found a really good way to get lots of glass in short order at "glass beach," climbed Ballyhoo on the wrong, steep side, lugged tons of junk back from Summer Bay, visited the docks, and conned a fresh opilio crab out of a crabber. It was delicious. Marlaine butchered it for us at the clinic. Marlaine knows how to do everything.

Ann made friends with Abi at Nicky's Place and came home with a loaf of Russian bread and the possibility of a skiff ride on Saturday. We had Marlaine, Chris (her boyfriend), and Clare over for fresh scallops Friday night. Dinner was fantastic, if I do say so myself. We all had a good time and they didn't leave until 11 or so.

I found out that Marlaine had been a rodeo rider as well as a nurse in Texas when she saw a want ad in the paper asking for ranch hands on the ranch in Chernofski on Unalaska Island. She was intrigued, quit her nursing job and came up here as a range rider on the sheep and cattle ranch. After a few years she found the opening for a nurse here at the clinic. Chris is a shipwright, among other things. He is funny, articulate and highly verbal.

Ann and I were up early on Saturday to get things done and be ready for the skiff ride, but the weather was too sloppy for the skiff so Abi drove us out to Morris Cove for beach-combing. We managed to get stuck in the mud even in four-wheel drive. It took us 10 minutes or so to push our way out. Fortunately the mud wasn't full of spawned-out salmon or we would have really stunk. We tried a different route after we got it out—we forded a stream on foot. I had to loan my boots to Ann. It was a real adventure, with great beachcomb-ing. We took pictures of each of us seated on the beach in a red-cushioned armchair that had washed ashore. Ann didn't find her glass float but we saw lots of shells and driftwood. Thence home with our loot. Abi stayed for drinks and dinner, though we didn't eat until about 11 p.m. She said we'd try the skiff on Sunday if the weather improved.

On Sunday Ann and I took the Padilla Tug 9 a.m. free trip to Hog Island in Unalaska Bay, just off the approach to the airstrip. We walked to the top and saw black rabbits and tons of rabbit poop plus two morel mushrooms. It was even better than beachcombing! Back at the beach we were really close to an eagle's nest. Mom and Pop were none too happy and screamed their disapproval but were nonetheless beauti-ful. On down the beach we saw a fresh seagull nest with three eggs. The eggs are shaped in such a way that they don't roll down the beach into the water. We ate our peanut-butter and pickle sandwiches, had hot tea, and met the boat a little after noon.

Once home we went down to Nicky's to meet Abi, and from there up to her home on Ski Bowl Road. (Her first one was a converted WW II barracks latrine.) We got gas, oars,

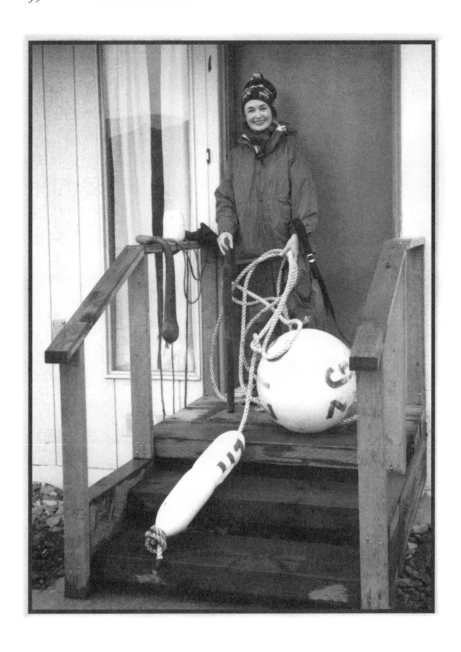

Sister ANN *after a day of beachcombing.*

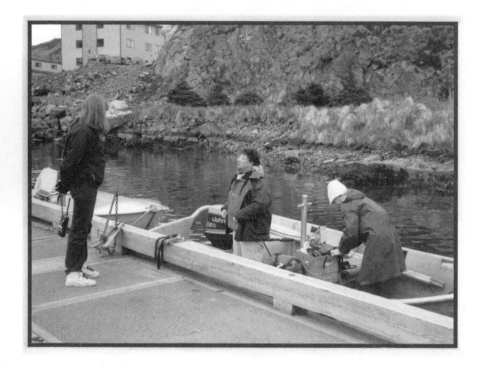

ABI *at the tiller,* NANCY *as passenger,* MARLAINE *conferring on the dock.*

etc., put our gear in a wheelbarrow and wheeled it out to the dock. We had bailed 50 or 60 gallons of water out of the skiff on Saturday so it was ready to go. It is a 14-foot Chignik-style seine skiff and reminds me of the wonderful Metlakatla dory our family had when we lived in Juneau. They both look, and are, very seaworthy. Abi's is ¼-inch-plate aluminum, flat-bottomed with skegs (downward pointing fins) on the bottom that cut through the water when the boat is going directly forward or in reverse. This little skiff is meant to pull the seine net closed when full of salmon—a purse seine—and the skegs keep it from side-slipping unless it is a deliberate slide to gain angle while pulling the net around the fish. There is a tow-bar amidship, and Abi has a 55-horse outboard motor with a stainless steel "work prop" on it, but the skiff still runs about 35 knots. She uses it to haul logs off the beach for firewood to heat her home. There are no trees in the Aleutians so people use what the tide brings them. Metalbestos chimneys, which usually last 25 years, will only go 10 here because of the salt in the wood.

We pushed off from the dock and wound lines around our arms to keep us on board. There were no life jackets. ("They just prolong the agony of dying," Abi says.) I balanced standing in the bow to help keep it down. I learned that sitting on the seat in even small seas would pound my spine so much that I would lose at least two inches of height. And what a trip we had!

Abi manned the tiller, taking us out past Summer Bay and Morris Cove to the edge of Constantine Bay, where on Lena Point, with its sheer rock cliff, we saw the remains of a concrete WW II lookout post. What a limited life those young men must have had. I couldn't imagine hauling the concrete and building materials up that rock face. Constantine Bay is broad and lovely, with gently sloping beaches. The shore is flat and we could see across the lake to Kalekta Bay, toward the Pacific side. We didn't go ashore because we knew if Ann got there we would never get her off. She loves to scavenge, which makes her home in Bellevue, Washington, more interesting than many museums. When she stayed with me at the townhouse she made a different centerpiece for the table every night.

The best was yet to come—Princess Cape. It is exactly that, a cape fit for royalty, which we felt by this time. It is an enormous columnar basalt formation covered with various lichens, making it appear a god-made mosaic. The light was just right, so it seemed spot-lit. Mystical. The water was "deep green flat" and the tide out a bit so it showed a base of mussels and kelp-strips of color to frame the cape as nothing else could. The swirls of basalt seemed to be folds of the cape, undulating gently to its base, all golds and greens and lacy white lichen. I am sure my camera failed to catch its grandeur.

I didn't want to leave but we had "miles to go." Next was the sea-cave, a black hole inhabited by young cormorants perched upon a ledge looking like water snakes in the gloom. We idled the entire boat into the cave and it gave us an eerie, claustrophobic feeling. The far end was completely dark, with the only visible thing the red eyes of the birds as the skiff rose and fell on the waves. Beneath us in the crystal clear water we were able to see huge boulders backlit by the sunlight coming from the mouth of the cave. Above us were deep spaces in the ceiling where the boulders had fallen out. Creepy to think of part of the ceiling falling out and landing in the skiff.

Still reeling from the sea cave and Princess Cape we went on to the corner of the bay and Outer Priest Rock, which really does look like a priest in black robes. It was impressive, but nothing to match the Cape. We pottered about while two rows of 14 inquisitive big-eyed seals watched, a regular gallery.

Sometimes when I am overwhelmed with the beauty of this place, I wonder how much the hard-working fishermen have time to see. From the patients I have treated I would guess that the ones with dollar signs for eyes don't see much else, but the others know how privileged they are. They seem to have an almost visible aura of joy and fulfillment about them.

Our next tack in the skiff was SW, passing Amaknak Island to the other side of Unalaska Bay. Boat motion was interesting, with the current running one way and the wind blowing the other. I have read where some boats go 40 to 60 miles offshore to avoid that kind of current out at Cape Kovrizhka, and here we were in a 14-foot skiff—but it has skegs, and Abi at the helm!

After running along the cliffs we saw the "outside" waterfall, which is hundreds of feet high, and then slipped back around the corner to Eider Point. The reef there is several thousand feet long and only a few feet deep on the ocean side. On the inside, strangely enough, in the bight, it plunges straight down into deep green nothingness. We tied up in some kelp and jigged unsuccessfully for sea bass. I would like to catch one sometime. Abi says they really fight and get to be over 100 years old. We finally beached inside the reef and

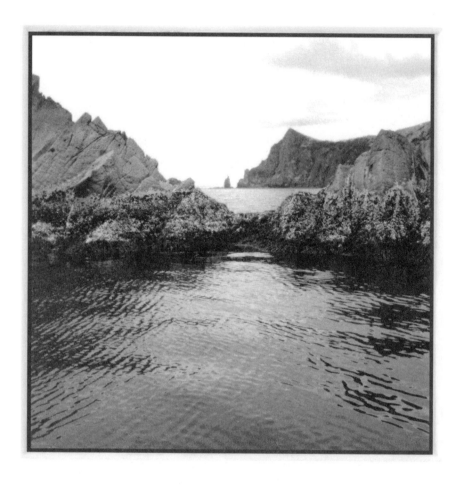

Looking out from PRINCESS CAPE *toward* PRIEST ROCK
in the far distance, center.

went to explore a fascinating old WW II sea-level lookout site positioned in the "crook" where the hill rolls down to the long curved spit. We ate lunch and sampled Abi's Edensoy, a soybean drink that tasted pretty good and really lasted, too. We didn't get hungry for hours. Good protein.

Moseying along the western shore to the "inside" waterfall we stopped at the jagged cliff that plunges straight down to the water. Abi tells us she has taken the skiff there and dropped anchor for an hour or two fishing for rock greenling (Steller's greenfish) or just watching marine life amongst the rocks and kelp. The greenling has interesting stripes and spines, but she says it is the turquoise flesh that boggles her. The first time she filleted one and cooked it she was horribly disappointed when the meat turned buff-colored. It was still tasty, but not exotic. The Natives call greenling "pogy" and use them for bait for black cod.

A puffin rookery sat above on the cliff, small but very active with puffins zooming around and buzz-bombing us while going into and out of their burrows, sometimes with as many as three candlefish in their mouths. How can a puffin catch and carry three at a time? How do they scoop up number three without numbers one and two getting loose?

On to Broad Bay, where there is good winter skiing in Makushin Valley, and then Nateekin Bay. There we went up the river, which is 20 feet wide at the mouth but much narrower farther up, where it varies in depth from 2 to 10 feet of clear water. Abi told us of all the plants that grow there. She says there may be as many as 15 types of orchids growing on Unalaska Island, and at times six to eight types in the tundra on that hillside. The whole trip was so impressive that it is

etched in my memory and I can go back and visit again and
again.

. .

March 19, 1992 — Tuesday.

Because this is a "one week" trip, it has been ultra busy,
with no time for anything but work. The weather has been
foul anyhow, and avalanches still block the road to Summer
Bay, so I guess it is just as well. The wind is blowing wet snow
sideways today, beating against the windows as I write.

I am in Clare's apartment this time. (I never know in
advance where I will be staying because it depends on who in
the clinic is on vacation.) The apartment is the new one 50
feet off the airport road—gorgeous view, but noisy with road
traffic. I would rather hear surf. Last trip out I stayed in her
old duplex on Standard Oil Hill where the feral cat jumped in
the window and onto my chest when I was sound asleep.
What an awakening! Especially because the front door to the
duplex would never actually close.

Tonight after work I had dinner at the Unisea Galley. It is
pleasant and the food is good. Not having to cook for myself
after a long day is a real plus. I drove down to the docks in
the clinic car past the *Mr. B* to look for birds and saw some
poor guy struggling through the storm with two heavy duffle-
bags. I thought of my son Ben, when he was out here all alone
with no place to stay out of the rain and wind while looking
for work, so stopped to see if he wanted a ride. Did he ever!
He had come up on a freighter because they said there were
"lots of jobs in Dutch." Naturally, there weren't, so he had
been living for five days in a 7×7×3-foot crab pot which he

had enough sense to cover with visqueen. Last night was so bad that he tried moving into an old abandoned brick building but found water everywhere. He had finally gotten a job on the *Royal Aleutian* and was moving his gear, so I took him there. He was one happy camper.

Tonight Marlaine is staying with me because she can't get up to her place on Ski Bowl Road with the roads slick with new snow. She is on call, and a patient with a compound leg fracture is supposed to be coming in at 2 a.m. I am glad I don't have to go.

Dr. Brockman, an orthopedist, has been here for several weeks. His presence is a real plus, with all the orthopedic injuries. He seems quite pleasant, and having another physician around is nice. I think he and I leave about the same time.

Other good news is from Milt and Cora Holmes, the owners of the sheep ranch at Chernofski, who have invited me out this summer. The ranch lies 85 miles southwest of here with headquarters on Mailboat Cove just inside Chernofski Harbor. The ranch is accessible only by sea. I can't imagine a sheep ranch of 152,000 acres in the Aleutians, but it has been there successfully since 1918. The main income is from wool, but meat is also sold to fishing boats as well as in the village of Unalaska. Milt must write wonderful ads—he managed to lure Marlaine from Texas and Cora, a pediatric intensive-care nurse from Idaho, to be a caretaker. After Cora had been working there for some time, she and Milt were married. Cora later lost her right hand to cancer and was fitted with a hook. She learned to spin yarn and weave using her left hand and the hook.

Marlaine says to see Stephanie Madsen about trying to catch a boat out there. Wouldn't that be fun? I would love it. It is time for bed. I am sure work will be sizzling tomorrow.

· ·

Oct. 15, 1992 — Tuesday.

WE WERE SO BUSY ALL SUMMER THAT I neglected my journal. I certainly would have written about the 50th anniversary in June of the WW II bombing of Dutch Harbor. The activities included a "Confederate Air Force" made up of pilots from the South who re-enacted the attack, using aircraft made to look like the real Zeros that actually did the bombing. Many of the men who had been here in 1942 were in town for the event, and I learned a lot about the defense of this vital place. The gun emplacement we saw at Eider Point on the wonderful skiff ride with Abi is just below a much larger one, the third of three such sites which together effectively blockaded the two entrances to Dutch Harbor. The one on the northwest side of Mt. Ballyhoo is the central and most extensive of the three. The smallest is on the right side of Iliuliuk Bay above Humpy Cove. Two submarine nets were to the south of the gun emplacements, one on Rocky Point to blockade Captain's Bay. The other, to blockade Iliuliuk Bay, extended from the spit near the original Dutch Harbor over to the shore near Summer Bay. No subs were ever in the harbor. Lacking room for a proper landing strip for planes, they rigged up a catapult and arrest system just like that used on aircraft carriers. This was done where the strip is now. (On some landings here I wish they still had an arrest system.)

My sister Ann was here with me again in June, and Cora and Milt were in town for the anniversary, so we flew back out with them in the Grumman Goose. The Goose got stuck on the beach but we unloaded and with everyone pushing managed to get the old girl back afloat. We in turn got weathered in and spent several wonderful days on the sheep ranch. I noticed that dear, thoughtful Milt had altered things in the kitchen to accommodate Cora's hook. We beach-combed (Ann found a glass ball right off), played Scrabble, went for walks, dug in mounds, had picnics, toured the slaughterhouse, carded wool, bottle-fed lambs, and loved every minute. I even found a beautiful 5½-inch bone harpoon head. Digging is legal there because the military has already screwed up the archeology and we were on private property. We had such a good time—Ann had her first flight in a Goose and I think she loved it. So did I. We will always have memories of the delightful kitchen and huge, wonderful cook-stove fired with coal from the WW II coal pile, of excellent food, and Cora and Milt with their parlor, the piano and library.

We departed for Dutch on a clear day, so Tom Madsen, a pilot of great renown, took us on a tour over different bays and burial mounds and through the mountains. We went on into Captain's Bay over Shaishnikoff Pass and then Dutch, where we landed on the water and crawled (waddled) up onto the tarmac.

· ·

THIS TRIP OUT [OCTOBER] HAS BEEN GREAT. IT IS my second tour to supervise Marlaine, who is better than I thought she would be and I always knew she would be good. It is a real

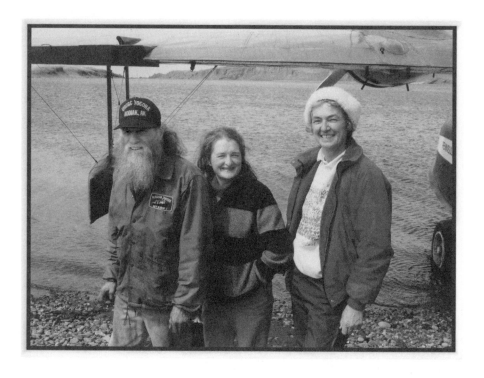

AT CHERNOFSKI *with* MILT *and* CORA HOLMES.

joy to have such a good pupil. The obstetrical protocol we have established includes the same lab work and visits at indicated intervals and even the same forms used in Anchorage. Marlaine is being trained to carry on when I leave. She really enjoys what she is doing and does it so well. Her school was excellent, and I have no doubt she will pass her boards. During the period I have been coming regularly the obstetrical load has more than quadrupled. Women aren't afraid to get pregnant out here any more. This gives me a very satisfying feeling. I think we did a good job.

Last trip Abi and her husband, Farid, took me up a road new to me that led to the main water reservoir at Icy Creek in Pyramid Valley. The creek was beautiful, with small falls and large pools of crystal-clear water, complete with "goldfins" (small gold-colored fish, probably trout). Marlaine told me of a creek before you come to Crowley Maritime, where in fall it is possible to walk up the creek bed to a spectacular double fall about half an hour away. I did that Tuesday night. I think I like the more tranquil falls better, but it was fun clambering about the rocks in near vertical canyons.

I have the use of the clinic car now when I come but because the tour is only Mon–Fri and I work such long hours there isn't time or energy to do much exploring. Maybe when I can come less often, as I expect in 1993, I'll extend over Saturday a couple of times in the summer. I've been at Pat's place the last two times and Jim's before that, so the walk to work doesn't take me near water where I can see all the sea life and birds. I miss that.

10-16-92

WEDNESDAY—NO ONE in Dutch is able to do vasectomies and I love to do them because I think it only fair for men to share the responsibility of parenthood. I talked the front desk into offering a "Vasectomy Special" over the radio. It always interests me how cautious patients in remote places are—understandable since they don't really get to know the various practitioners. I had a mental picture of all the guys down at the Elbow Room (local bar) shooting dice to see who would go first. The predictable test patient came for his vasectomy and I could tell how nervous he was, but everything went very well. When he had successfully healed and was still in one piece (though minus a bit) the phone started ringing for the Special. I think we have done five more since then. I enjoyed being able to provide a service otherwise unavailable.

Pat's "alarm cat" got me up at 6 today, poor lonely thing. No wind or rain so it must be foggy. Feels like early fall in Lynden, Washington, where I grew up. I love the quiet of this place. It is time to clean the house and get ready to leave. Pat will be back when I come next month and the cat can get back to a normal life after having endless itinerants caring for it in her absence.

· ·

March 11, 1993 — Thursday.

THE STAFF MOVED INTO THE NEW CLINIC building in December and had the official open house Feb. 14. Certainly more spacious than the old clinic but no more efficient, and the room Marlaine and I use is too small by far. A real pain for colposcopy (a colposcope is a big microscope on wheels used to examine the mouth of the uterus to look for abnormalities found on the Pap smear) and I hope I never have to do a vasectomy there. It is better than the old place, though. The waiting room must seem heaven to the patients. They have also added real lab techs on a rotating basis. I really like the one who is here now. She knows her stuff.

On all my trips since January I have been quartered in the two-bedroom doctor's apartment here in this new building. Ron Brockman, the orthopedist, shares it with me (after assuring me that he didn't "sleepwalk" at night). The clinic was going to furnish it with cast-offs from the town, but Ron bought all new furniture for it because he is spending five to six months at a time here. With the huge amount of orthopedic trauma in the fishing industry, his presence is a blessing. The apartment is complete with CD player, TV and VCR, a kitchen and small living room. We spent off-time during my January rotation putting furniture together.

While the view is of the hillside mere inches away, the apartment is as quiet as anywhere I have stayed while here. Because I have been leaving my cello here in the clinic, I go down to the conference room on the other end of the building to practice. The "break room" is across the hall from my room. The NordicTrack I bought the clinic is there so everyone can use it. It is great to look out at the harbor and "ski" away. I imagine I am on the road to Summer Bay.

It was an easy trip in, and I got to go up in the cockpit for a while. But we had a terrible storm the night we got here. Wind so bad it even shook my bed, and this is a huge building. It snowed, too. Marlaine said they had six-foot drifts.

When I got up on Tuesday it was gorgeous as only the Aleutians can be—brilliant sun reflected off the new snow and the bay as quiet as if it were painted. I went from window to window all day, gaping. I took a long walk after dinner, cold, but beautiful. And then Wednesday was the same!

In an impulse I understood very well, Collette and Tiny called for a barbecue on the beach. Reminds me of spring picnics Syd and I would have at Sand Lake in Anchorage when it was sunny, all of us in coats and parkas sitting next to a snow bank and drinking champagne.

"Come join us on Little South America," they said.

"Little South America?"

"Yeah, in Chile, above Tierra Del Fuego."

Were they nuts? No, it seems that the southern tip of Amaknak Island is shaped like South America and everyone in town knows all the places that are relevant. "Bunker Hill," which is on the right coming from the airport just before the Bridge to the Other Side, is in Venezuela. The Pacific side of Little South America is part of Captain's Bay. The Atlantic side faces the South Channel between Amaknak and Unalaska islands.

Clare picked me up with a jug of her homemade beer under her arm and we drove to Little South America, above Tierra Del Fuego. Tiny and his pards had stacks of pallet boards from which they were feeding a large bonfire. It felt good against the cold breeze off the water. Tiny also had a huge 5- or 10-gallon pot of beans on a propane burner ordinarily used for cooking crab. Next to it was a charcoal burner for hamburgers.

Someone brought a whole pickup full of chips and dips. Then another bunch of folks drove in with a big barrel cooker, a 55-gallon oil drum cut in half lengthwise. With a grill laid across it, they cooked chicken and more hamburgers. Lots of dogs were hanging around, and kids too, some sledding in the hills just above the beach. Radio on loud. A big sea lion cruised along just off shore and stopped to look us over. One or two boats puttered past. As it got darker the stars came out in that clearest of skies. Every time someone threw another pallet board on the fire we saw our own Milky Way of fiery red sparks swirling upward. It was better than the Fourth of July.

The group was a comfortable one, a lot like the crab-feed parties we used to have in Juneau. Marlaine and her boyfriend, Chris, were both having a good time. We stuffed ourselves on hamburgers with bleu cheese, barbecued chicken, teriyaki chicken, and Tiny's fantastic beans. Hours later the last pallet went on the fire and we trudged through the mud under that crystal canopy of stars to return to the real world of Dutch Harbor and mud-encrusted trucks.

▪ ▪

How RARE TO HAVE such a run of beautiful days! Today is brilliant as the previous ones. Tiny wanted me to see his new clay pigeon launcher so he and Collette invited Bruce, one of the clinic PA's, and me up for trap shooting and dinner. We drove up yet another road I didn't know existed. Turns out to be the one to Beaver Inlet—well, not quite, but it goes up to the crest and then on down to Summer Bay. Tiny pulled off and set up the thrower. Zack has an Ithaca 12-gauge pump like mine. It is too long in the stock for me, but not bad. He is really good with it, as was Tiny with his "boat gun." Bruce and I were equally bad, but it was fun and I wasn't skunked entirely. The weather is cold and windy up there, which makes me think we are at the end of this stretch of nice weather. We had a good dinner of chicken tetrazzini in their geodesic dome house. Tiny said the company he works for paid $250,000 for the house and three-quarter acre of land. I nearly fainted at the magnitude of the price. It sure is nicer than their old house on Standard Oil Hill. They are obviously pleased with the life they have worked so hard to attain. (Later I learned that the previous owner of their new property was returning from Anchorage on a Mark Air plane in rough weather when they dragged a wing on landing and crashed, tearing off an engine—the same crash I had heard about. He managed to get out and ended up in a dazed condition on the runway, surrounded by gallons of jet fuel which fortunately did not ignite. He had had enough, so he quit his job and he and his family moved out, leaving the house for sale.)

. .

I THINK THE GREAT bottom fishery here has begun to dry up. Gluttony has once again killed the fish that laid the golden eggs. There certainly aren't nearly as many patients here this year as there were two years ago. I'm glad to have been here during the boom years but I won't be sad to see it smaller, with fewer oil slicks and less slurry on the bottom and filth on the beaches.

I saw Cora in the airport going out as I was coming in. Mark Air now has a mail run out past their ranch in Chernofski and it will stop there for $87 each way from Dutch. Maybe Ann and I will go out there for a while in May on my last trip out here. We shall see. I would like to be in Chernofski again.

. .

MY SHOJI SCREEN ARRIVED! I suppose I should explain this great event. In Anchorage I belong to a woodworking club and do quite a bit in my spare time. Every February during Fur Rendezvous there is a competition in woodworking where we all display what we have made during the year (or two or three). Of all the various classes—furniture, wood carving, boxes, turning—one of the most interesting is "See what you can make out of an 8-foot piece of green Alaska Birch." The results are wondrous. People make everything from children's toys to lamps. I made a music stand using bent lamination a few years ago and enjoyed it, so this year I decided to make a shoji screen using bent lamination for the interior design of kimoko. I had no real use for one and planned to put it in the show and afterward have a party for my friends and burn it in a bonfire. It turned out much better than I had expected. It was such a pleasure to watch people come into the room, see my shoji and say, "Oh, look at that, it's so beautiful"—and I won first prize so there was no bonfire. It sat at home on its two little feet awaiting destiny.

When the clinic was in the planning stages they asked all of us to view the plans and make comments. I could see that all the doors to the examining rooms opened on the wrong side, so that when the door to the room was opened the partially clothed patient on the examining table would be exposed to everyone in the hall. I pointed out this problem but no one listened, and the doors do indeed give a great view to anyone passing by. Aha! I have an unused shoji screen just the right size for the room Marlaine and I use. But how to get it safely out here with its fragile rice-paper backing and the thin laminated design within the frame?

Janice Reeve Ogle is a flight attendant on the family planes (Reeve Aleutian Airways) and a former patient of mine in my Anchorage practice. In the early days of my trips to Dutch she once had a birthday party for me on the plane, complete with a gift of a Reeve carry-on bag and a Reeve book plus coffee and cake and the passengers singing "Happy Birthday." I called her and explained my problem. She said she would baby-sit the screen on the flight, keeping it safe from the jaws of the forklift and last-minute bags being thrown in. It has arrived in perfect condition and Marlaine is pleased with it. It looks as if it were made for the room and will shield the patients very well. I'm going to take my camera along next time and take a picture of Marlaine at her desk with her son's Southwest Indian art on the wall behind her and the screen to her right. So far no one has poked a hole in it.

Ron went sea bass fishing last Sunday. After they had caught some, they saw a dolphin and then were suddenly surrounded by hundreds of them, leaping and playing. I saw his video and it is wonderful. Three and four out of the water at once, like chariot horses, with all kinds of them in the background. Water so clear they could be seen playing at the bow as the boat moved.

Time to fold. Up early in the morning to pack and get all the linens washed. Naturally I will use the NordicTrack and shower and wash my hair first—oh, yeah!

. .

May 1993 — My last tour of duty for the Iliuliuk Clinic.

My job here is done, with a good obstetrical protocol in place. Marlaine is well trained to carry it on. I plan to have uninterrupted time at home once again, with season tickets to the symphony, classes at UAA, playing cello in the Civic Orchestra and building things in my garage.

Clinic staff has planned a farewell party for me upstairs in the Shishaldin Room at the Grand Aleutian Hotel. Neither the hotel nor the present clinic was in existence when I started coming here. How very rewarding it is to see the improvement in the quality of medical care and at least an interest in improving the working conditions of everyone in the fishing industry, with its current excessive incidence of injury.

I will miss the wild beauty of this place and the palpable energy that strikes me every time I step off the plane. So, too, will I miss the diversity of the people who live here. I will miss their intensity, their love of what they are doing, and their ability to cope under trying circumstances. I have always thought it important to be a participant rather than an observer in life, and every person I have met out here is an ardent participant.

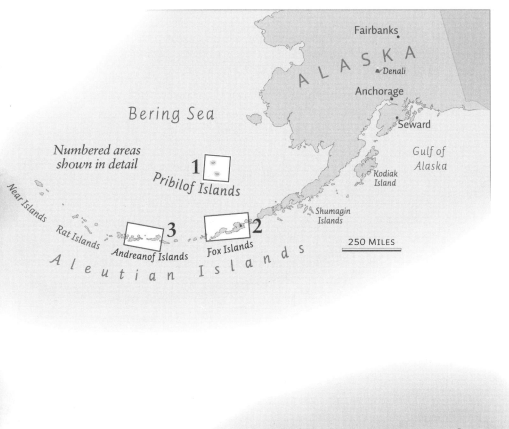

Fairbanks

A L A S K A

Denali

Anchorage

Bering Sea

Seward

Gulf of
Alaska

Numbered areas
shown in detail

1

Pribilof Islands

Kodiak
Island

Shumagin
Islands

Near Islands

Rat Islands

3

2

250 MILES

Andreanof Islands

Fox Islands

A l e u t i a n   I s l a n d s

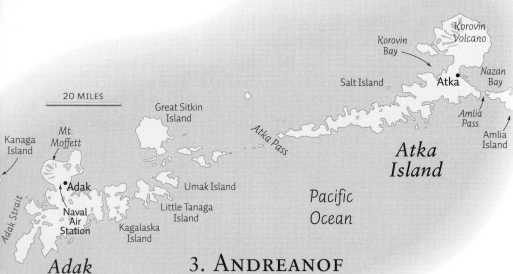

Korovin
Volcano

Korovin
Bay

Salt Island

Atka

Nazan
Bay

20 MILES

Great Sitkin
Island

Atka Pass

Amlia
Pass

Amlia
Island

Kanaga
Island

Mt.
Moffett

Atka
Island

Adak

Umak Island

Pacific
Ocean

Adak Strait

Naval
Air
Station

Little Tanaga
Island

Kagalaska
Island

Adak
Island

3. ANDREANOF
ISLANDS

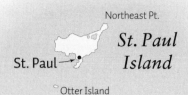

Northeast Pt.

*St. Paul
Island*

St. Paul →

Otter Island

1. PRIBILOF
ISLANDS

Dalnoi Pt.   **St. George**

*St. George
Island*

20 MILES

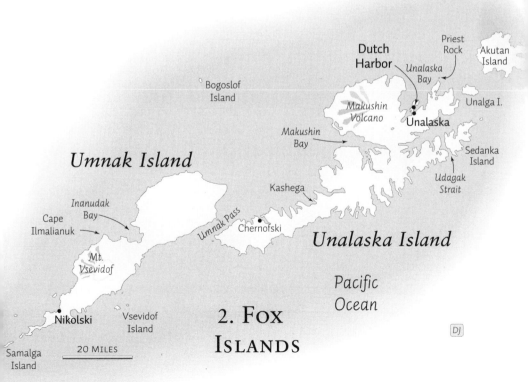

Priest
Rock

Akutan
Island

**Dutch
Harbor**

*Unalaska
Bay*

Bogoslof
Island

*Makushin
Volcano*

Unalga I.

Unalaska

*Makushin
Bay* →

Sedanka
Island

Umnak Island

*Udagak
Strait*

Kashega

*Inanudak
Bay*

Umnak Pass

Cape
Ilmalianuk →

Chernofski

Unalaska Island

*Mt.
Vsevidof*

*Pacific
Ocean*

Nikolski   Vsevidof
Island

2. FOX
ISLANDS

DJ

Samalga
Island   20 MILES

"People come and they say, that's in the middle
of nowhere. But really it's in the middle of it all."

—*Aquilina Lestenkof of St. Paul,*
in People of the Seal: Pribilof Islands, Alaska

PART II

. .

Aleutian/Pribilof Islands Association

Ice Pack in the Pribilofs

Cold brushes my cheeks as I walk to the cliff above Bachelor Beach to watch the ice pack come in, bringing isolation until spring. The inner harbor has been solid for several days, with the pilot boat frantically crashing through the ice to make channels. Crabbers rush to off-load their catch before scurrying south to home ports and safety.

For once it is calm, and the mist rises thick and swirling from the open water near shore. Ice crystals tat themselves in lacy patterns across the turquoise water as it lifts and falls. The beach, once vibrant with seal voices, is now an empty concert hall after a stellar performance. The sea surges against the base of my cliff while the pack approaches warily from the north, its white teeth barely visible through sea smoke in the pale arctic light. The island is being stalked.

Across the water comes the faint chatter of bergs conversing in comfortable abrasion. Now the reticular surface patterns coalesce into a semi-solid sheen and the chatter deepens to a thrum of tension between great forces as the pack moves in. Then silence—

On my cliff, I am a lone foxfire at the changing tree, readying myself for this winter season.

—N.E.S.

NOT LONG AFTER THE FAREWELL PARTY IN UNALASKA, I received a call from the Aleutian/Pribilof Islands Association (APIA), a not-for-profit Native corporation for which I had already made several trips to St. Paul. Now they asked if I would be interested in working as an itinerant to their other islands as well—the Pribilofs, plus Unalaska, which is nearest to Anchorage, and Umnak, Atka, and Adak, all farther west.

I knew of the wonderful "Pribs," St. George and St. Paul, with their enormous seal population, and I had heard the story of their discovery by an Aleut man named *Igiadax*. He set out from Unalaska in his *iqyax* (kayak) and was caught by a monstrous storm and blown 250 miles to the north, where he finally made it ashore. How long does it take to travel 250 miles in a kayak? Not very long if the winds are 90 miles per hour. But what if the seas are over 50 feet? What does that feel like? When he landed he was amazed to see the entire beach covered with seals. Everywhere he looked—seals and more seals. He thought he had blown ashore on seal heaven, where seals went when they died.

And how did this man, having been blown 250 miles to a place he had never been and did not know existed, find his way home? No compass, no GPS, no motor, no sail, no map, no radio, no satellite phone—he just paddled back the way he had come. I continue to have tremendous respect and admiration for these seafarers, the Aleuts.

My travels, I assumed, would be a little less adventurous. Itinerant meant I was to go when needed, where needed, among the islands. The villages ranged in population from 32 to several hundred people, and the work varied accordingly, with fishing ports having the highest number of trauma cases. St. Paul and Unalaska were the two fishing ports, but they had the luxury of at least one PA or NP (physician's assistant or nurse practitioner) with whom to trade being on call.

· ·

IN UNALASKA, MY OLD ILIULIUK CLINIC WAS now on the first floor in a new building. The Oonalaska Wellness Center, APIA's clinic, was on the second floor, with access up the small hill from the clinic parking lot. By 1993, the Iliuliuk Clinic had hired permanent lab techs and two fulltime doctors, who would provide back-up in difficult cases. In all the other villages it was to be a solo role. I would give the shots, do the lab, start the IV, take the x-ray, call for medivac and care for the patient until help arrived by way of Coast Guard C-130 out of Kodiak or one of the medivac teams from Anchorage. Either option was three to four hours distant in the best of weather, and often delayed a day or more.

For consults the PA's or I could call appropriate doctors at the Alaska Native Medical Center in Anchorage. They were already working as hard and fast as possible, so replies were often some time in coming. Several years ago "telemed" was initiated and was a tremendous help, when the weather didn't take out the antenna or the receiver. With telemed we could often manage to keep patients on the island instead of having them make the arduous and expensive trip to town for a consult. We could write a brief history, include any lab work or x-rays and even actual photographs, and send it all in for advice, which would come when the doctor at ANMC had time to check the telemed.

Getting from Anchorage to Umnak Island or to Atka or Adak meant not just one but two exciting flights, landing first at Dutch Harbor and then changing to a smaller plane to reach my assignment. Even if I managed to get in to Dutch I would often wait hours or days for weather to clear there or on the island I was headed to.

My favorite plane was the amphibian Grumman Goose, which flew to Chernofski Ranch on Unalaska Island and to Nikolski on Umnak. There are no roads to any of these villages. As in the Bush, transport is by boat or air. That old Goose would take off on wheels at Dutch, land on water at Chernofski, and waddle up onto the beach. At Nikolski in particular the Goose had a great advantage: If the wind was bad for the strip—where a crashed DC-3 still sat as a reminder of the difficulty—the pilot could simply land on the nearby lake with no trouble.

One of the joys of small planes for me as a private pilot was that I often got to sit in the co-pilot's seat. (Not very joyful if the plane iced up. I was so much more aware of that up front than I was sitting farther back. If the pilot seemed relaxed, I tried not to get anxious.)

Getting in to Atka was almost always exciting. I can't remember any arrival not involving let-down through low-lying clouds as the pilot threaded the plane through unseen but solid mountains. The airstrip is in a little valley out near the new village. I was always thrilled to break out of clouds and find us within sight of the strip, wedged between the mountains. (The clinic was in the old village on Nazan Bay, which is quite long and on the Pacific side of this island. They were in the process of making a new village over toward the narrow neck of land between Korovin Bay and Nazan Bay where the landing strip is.)

Atka village was charming for many reasons. It held only 80 to 90 people and was the one village I visited where Aleut was the

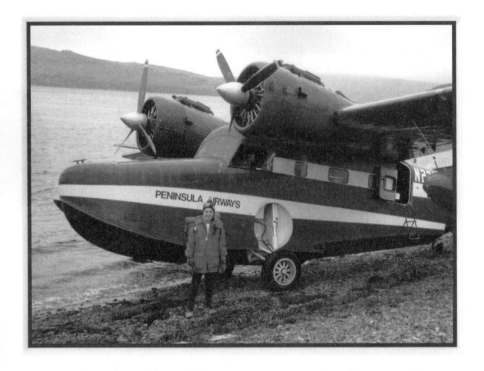

ANN *poses with the Grumman* GOOSE, *our favorite plane.*

spoken language. I was busy in the clinic one day when several people came running in, calling, "Doctor, doctor, come quick!" This was followed by a flow of Aleut. Before I could reach for the emergency bag, they grabbed me, pushed me onto a 4-wheeler, and took off flying down the road, rattling excited Aleut in my ear. "What can I do without my tools?" I wondered, as my mind rushed through the possibilities. Suddenly we stopped on the hill outside town, and there before us were reindeer! This time, in English, they said, "You see? They have come to offer themselves!" A few days later I was invited to share a wonderful roast. Millie Prokopeuff, who had the office next to mine in the clinic and held down two jobs, turned out to be a very good cook as well, which I learned when she invited me to share that feast.

· ·

THE ATKA CLINIC OCCUPIES the entire first floor of a building in the old village that is shared with the city government. The waiting room has two or three chairs plus the ever-present coffeepot. At first when I saw a full waiting room I worried about keeping patients waiting. Then I found that they just came to visit and drink coffee. A very pleasant custom.

Complete with a desk, filing cabinets, phones and a new computer, the office is what I call a "one-ass" office. I can reach everything in the room from my chair.

The hallway extends to the left from the office. Next to my office is Millie's. What a blessing she is, with answers to all my questions! Making travel arrangements for patients would be a nightmare without her assistance. (I see I have slipped into present tense. Describing it is almost as good as being there.)

A bathroom is on the right, then a small lab and supply room. Two exam rooms are on the left; at the end of the hall is a door where the ambulance can back in to deliver patients when necessary. The furnace room is just to the right of this door. Storage is a problem in most clinics; here there is a shed near both the ambulance entrance and the clinic entrance.

Quarters are above the clinic, across the hall from the city office —two bedrooms, a bath and a combination kitchen/living room. Because there are no hotels or inns in the village the second bedroom is rented out when needed. The view from the quarters is a hillside 10 feet away, but the view from the city office window is over the old village and across Nazan Bay. The door to the office had a large window as well; if I hankered for a view of the sea when the office was closed, I would open my door, stand in the hall, and get the view through the two office windows. When the fog lifted it was always beautiful, and soothing.

Boats bring rats, so any village involved with commercial fishing is soon plagued by them. The rats in Atka were so emboldened that they invaded the clinic on occasion. The fire escapes for the second-floor quarters consisted of ladders nailed to the wall below the windows. I like to sleep with open windows, and screens were often absent, so the "rat ladders" became a problem. I solved this by taking my black Labrador, Vita, with me to Atka. She was not only wonderful at hunting ptarmigan but valiant on the rat front.

. .

Vita and I had other adventures. Duck hunting was good on Atka, so we set off with the 4-wheeler early one morning with ducks in mind. Out past the landing strip was a lagoon and beyond that a stream that looked promising. (I was on call 24 hours a day on the island. On days that the clinic was closed I always phoned the local police to tell them where I was going and what time I expected to return, and I carried a two-way radio so I could be contacted in case of an emergency.) I parked the 4-wheeler, pulled my hip boots up, and shrugged into my pack loaded with extra shells, the transmitter for Vita's collar, and the radio. Shotgun in hand, Vita at heel, we set off.

As we neared the stream a flock of ducks flew up and I shot one, which fell into the stream. Vita dashed after it. When I got to the stream I discovered that the bank was almost perpendicular and at least five feet high above the water on both sides. Vita could not get out. I tried hanging onto bushes in order to reach for her but could not get close enough. Then I searched along the edge for a possible landing area—again, no luck. Vita is in good shape so was still swimming against the rapid flow and not being swept out into the bay, on the Bering Sea side of the island. I finally put my gun down, lay on my stomach with toes dug in for traction, and reached farther than before. What a mistake! It was too steep, and I did a somersault into the creek. Vita was glad to see me, and I at least managed to boost her up enough so she could scramble out.

Now our positions were reversed. I tried repeatedly with no success. I thought I might make it if I got rid of the weight of my pack, so I contrived to throw it up onto the bank, after which I thought, "That was smart! Now if you can't get out you can't call anyone for help!" I thought I might make it out if I could get my boots off. While struggling to accomplish this I floated downstream and noticed some well-rooted bushes that might hold my weight—and they did. I sloshed back along the bank, got my gun, the bird, and the pack, and we headed for the 4-wheeler and home. Vita kept warm by her favorite activity, running. I took a hot shower as soon as we got there.

. .

NIKOLSKI ON UMNAK ISLAND, THE NEXT ISLAND to the west from Unalaska, is such a beautiful village that I want my ashes spread there when I die. It was inhabited before the pyramids were built and I understand why. It has everything needed to sustain life: fish, berries, seal, and sea lion—all in a wondrous setting in the shadow of Mt. Vsevidof, 13 miles distant. Even now when I close my eyes I can see the crescent of the harbor with its reefs and Anangula Island to the right, next to Okee Point, and on the left, Coast Guard Bay and its glorious tide pools full of brilliant life.

Ah, the tide pools! Once when I was in Nikolski the word went around that the elders were hankering for "gumboots" (chiton). Great, I thought, now I can do something for them. I love tide pools and knew where the chiton slept on a sort of underwater cliff, slippery and difficult to reach. I had photographed those impressive pools so was sure where to go. Alternately sliding and crawling, I made it out onto the reef at low tide and gathered a sack full—an invigorating afternoon. Then I distributed the chiton to the elders, much to their joy and mine. I asked how they prepared gumboots for eating and they just laughed and said, "Gumboots are good raw." I had some left and decided to emulate the elders. "Gumboots" was a good name. They were sort of chewy, but I didn't mind—I was so proud of myself. In the middle of the night, though, my stomach rebelled. Alas, I learned that unlike oysters on the half-shell, the only edible part of a gumboot is the "foot." I'm still glad for the gathering, though.

Nikolski had 30-some residents when I worked there. Sadly, that number has declined to perhaps two dozen people as this is written. Population decline is common in any village changing from a subsistence lifestyle to a cash economy. This requires houses rather than barabaras, furnaces in place of driftwood, and grocery stores instead of the shared bounty of the surroundings. There are other complex issues but this seems to be the main one. A hunting and fishing lodge was built in an effort to employ more local people. It offers halibut fishing and duck hunting among other opportunities, but the weather often makes it difficult to get to or from the island. Most hunters from the mainland don't want to wait a week or more in Dutch trying to get there when they have only a week to hunt. The lodge seemed an excellent idea, but not many clients have come, and the population continues to decline.

Entering the clinic at Nikolski, in one of the small HUD houses built after World War II, is like entering a typical home, with an entry hall for coats and boots. The living room/kitchen, which is now a waiting room/office, is to the right, with a wood stove, useful when the furnace goes out. Large windows in the living room area give a beautiful view of Vsevidof. The opposite windows, in the kitchen area, look toward a neighboring house and the Russian Orthodox church.

A hall reached by either the entry or the kitchen has a furnace room on the left and a bathroom on the right. At the end of the hall is an exam room on the left and a storage room on the right, with a cot for the CHA or me. There is no lab or x-ray equipment, and no laundry facilities. I always think of this as a "house" and not a "clinic" and refer to it as such in my journals.

. .

St. Paul and St. George, the Pribilof Islands, are farther north and require a different routing from Anchorage. Sometimes the plane would go via Dutch Harbor, but usually it stopped for gas in King Salmon, Dillingham or Cold Bay.

St. George Island is slightly larger (about 12 by 5 miles) than St. Paul (about 10 by 5 miles), but it has a much smaller population—around 100 people—and unlike St. Paul is not a fishing port with processors. There is no real harbor on St. George, and it was amusing to see the tour boats anchor out in the sea and send birdwatchers and tourists via open skiff to the small dock in the village. The water is so shallow that the baby seals are taught to swim there. The only major access to St. George is by air, and the strip on the opposite side of the island is frequently plagued by fierce crosswinds.

The clinic building is a relatively new one-story structure, with the clinic on one side and the quarters on the other. In the waiting room, as in most clinics, are a few chairs and a coffeepot plus hot water for tea. On the left as one enters is a room for the health aide (or me), and beyond it a fairly large room that holds supplies and a drug refrigerator. On the right from the entrance is a hall leading first to a room filled with telemed equipment and then to an exam room, which connects to the ER farther back. Between the two rooms is a short hall with a bathroom on the right and a supply closet on the left. The ER has two work stations, but it would be difficult to deal with more than one patient at a time because the room is so crowded with equipment.

The last room on the right is a small lab used mainly for blood-draw equipment and mailing supplies for sending samples to Anchorage. The door to the outside is at the end of the hall. Opposite the lab are a janitor's room and the x-ray room.

The quarters in the other half of the building are entered via either the waiting room or an outside door at the far end of the building. Entering from the waiting room, the bedroom with bath is on the left (and quite spacious, with a clothes closet and room for a desk at the end of the bed). A hall leads from the bedroom door to the living/dining room, which has both a table and a davenport. The windows look out across the village. On entering, the kitchen is to the left of the living room, with refrigerator, freezer, range, and microwave. At the far end of the living room is another short hall leading to the outside door, past the furnace room on the left.

When I first went to St. George there was no TV or computer access. Now there are both, at the clinic and at the Aikow Inn—when the wind hasn't blown the antennas away.

• •

MY FIRST VISIT TO ST PAUL, THE northernmost island of the Pribilofs, was in the spring of 1991. Passengers disembarked down the plane steps onto the apron, walked 30 yards or so into the hangar, and then proceeded up a ramp on one side through some doors into the waiting room. I did not pick up luggage here because Reeve trucked it all to a warehouse downtown. I was met by one of the ex-navy medics, who drove me to town in a well-worn Chevy truck that belonged to the clinic. He pointed out the luggage pick-up site, which was in the back of A/C (Alaska Commercial), the general store only a block or so from the clinic.

The clinic is a long white two-story building just past the King Eider Hotel, the only inn on the island. The medic showed me the way to my clinic quarters through an outside door next to the King Eider. I entered a comfortable living/dining room and then proceeded down a hall past two bedrooms and a bath. We went through yet another door into a hall that led to the clinic. In a few steps we passed the clinic "break room" on the left, and thence into the back hall of the clinic, running between the ER and the lab and ambulance entrance on the right. The ER appeared to be well-equipped. I was delighted to think that I wouldn't have to go outside in the weather to get to the clinic when I was on night call. Most convenient—if I didn't get lost in that maze.

The medic explained that the building was an old TB hospital built in the 1920s. The clinic now occupied the entire first floor; the second floor was used by dentists and mental health personnel. We proceeded down the hall to the medic's office, with a recovery room on the right and then three exam rooms. On the left were a bathroom, a janitor's room, the x-ray room and a door to the basement (one I would use often in the future to adjust the wayward furnace and to do laundry).

Just past this door was the front office and the waiting room, both of which were accessible from the enclosed porch on that end of the building. The medical offices were to the right of the front desk, and as soon as we reached it I was put to work. It was very similar to the work in Unalaska, with the same joys and hazards.

Because there were three of us I could have an occasional day off to explore the island, and I had the Chevy to do it in. Ah, the beautiful beaches miles long, the seals, the birds on the cliffs, the reefs, the foxes! *Igiadax* had it right: It is heaven for seals, and for us, too.

Later in the summer of 1991, a few months after my sister Ann's husband had died, she came out to the island with her friend Betty Lane. There were bunk beds in the second bedroom in quarters, so they stayed with me and explored the island while I worked. And work the aides and I did! I was so busy that I didn't have time to keep a journal. I do have a picture of Ann in her red parka hiking down a very empty, long and gorgeous beach all alone. I love the picture because to me it told so much of Ann and where she was in life, plus what she was doing about it.

St. Paul

Oct 19, 1992—Monday.

REGGIE, MY BOSS AT APIA, AND I ALMOST didn't get out of Dutch in time to come to St. Paul. The fog was down to the deck. Good old Reeve held for about an hour or so over Dutch; when the fog cleared, the pilot popped the plane onto the strip and got out before the fog had a chance to return. It is an absolutely stunning day here. Cold, clear and windy—the usual 30–40-knot cross-wind on the runway. I had a window seat so got to see all the mountains and bays on the way out. Again, beautiful as only the Aleutians can be. I really want to follow a flight map sometime so I can figure out just where I am.

I love the efficiency of our leaders. We are here for only 48 hours and have arrived on a holiday so the clinic is closed. In addition, one-half the population is in Anchorage for the AFN (Alaska Federation of Natives) conference. I have a feeling this won't be a very productive trip. I was met by the clinic PA with the new Dodge Ram that is strictly for business because some yo-yo stuck the old Chevy royally and ruined the tranny. He had to be hauled out and then had the nerve to send the bill to the clinic! I note the Ram has only 145.7 miles on it, and it was here in summer when I came.

This time we are in the east end in rooms above the clinic that I didn't even know existed. I enter from a door in the clinic entry porch. Cold as usual for rooms here, and I am wearing a down vest while sitting next to a portable radiator. I see there is a hot water bottle here. Reggie and I will have to fight over it. None of the windows open and the bathroom sink is unusable. Other than that—

Reggie had a closet to sleep in the last time she was here, so I made her take the big sunny room on the east end. She did so with alacrity. I will bunk on the davenport in the living room.

After picking our luggage up at Reeve, we went for a walk. I had expected all the seals and sea lions to be gone but I guess they haven't left yet. There were many of them in the lee on Bachelor Beach. Reggie and I walked around and then split up because she needs time alone and I like to walk more and faster. I went out to the near rookery and was amazed to see the beach covered with seals. All the birds except seagulls are gone, though, leaving the cliffs bare and quiet. Lots of seals were playing in the surf so I sat down out of the wind to watch and soak up the surf sounds plus the changing hues of the sea. Sure beats TV. Was lazily lounging when I thought I saw a whale—sure enough, it was a small killer whale quite close to my cliff. Soon it was joined by another small one and then a full-sized one and then a super-sized one. All four fed back and forth in front of the cliff. They acted like the dolphins they are—just up and down over the surface of the water, which was so clear that I could see them even under water. I am sure they were looking for baby seals, on which they love to feed. They finally moseyed on up the coast. The liquidity and effortlessness of their movement is a joy to see. I feel very privileged.

It reminds me of that wonderful moment at Cold Bay a few years ago on a very windy goose hunt with my sons Bruce and Elliott. Elliott wanted to stay out and hunt although it was blowing 70 knots. It was the third day of the hunt and I was very tired. It had been a long, difficult walk for this old lady. Elliott had brought his own dog, so I decided to take my dog, Tigger, and trek on up to a little hill at the end of the lake we were hunting, between salt water and the lake. When we got there I settled to leeward just below the crest. I sat in delicious-smelling heather, completely protected from the wind in a hollow with my feet up as though I were in a chaise-lounge, and Tig was lying down as well. It was pure heaven—the softness, the protection from the wind, the smell and the position. Then I heard geese coming—emperors, who make that funny distinctive cackling. We sat still and here came a flock of 16 or 18 just over our heads! I could have reached up and grabbed them by the legs! It was truly wondrous. I enjoy being a part of it all and not just looking at pictures.

The water bottle needs to be heated. I'll get my bed warm and then let Reggie have the bottle for her bed.

Jan. 24, 1995 — Tuesday.

TRAVEL TIME WAS TWO DAYS TO GET to St Paul Island from Anchorage. I was scheduled to leave yesterday, the 23rd, so I got up at 5:30 a.m., packed a large cooler of frozen foods, my cello and music, a big duffle bag of clothing, books, music tapes and CD's plus a player, and loaded it all into a taxi. At the airport I sat drinking coffee and working the crossword puzzle in the paper for an hour while awaiting my fate. I was not confirmed on the flight, but flying "space available" on the wait list with quite a few others. Chances didn't look too good for getting on—and they weren't. What a shame—that flight made it all the way to St. Paul without being turned back by weather. Oh, well. I lugged all my gear back out to the taxi stand and went home to try again today—and I got here!

As we deplaned I met Jean Snow, a public health nurse who is to be my roommate for a few days. She is doing follow-up on all the tuberculosis cases while I will be sharing call with David Davelos, a PA-C (certified physician's assistant), one of the best PA's I ever worked with. We two will do all the general medicine for the village as well as care for the thousands of fishermen from the fleet and the processors.

The usual St. Paul ground blizzard greeted us on our arrival, and we crawled to town in the clinic truck with our luggage in the back. I used to think it had to be snowing to have a blizzard. I was wrong. Here in the "Birthplace of the Winds," if there is snow on the ground the wind just picks it up and throws it so thick I can't see two feet unless I were to manage very tall stilts in that wind. And then, although my head would be above it, all I could see would be a sea of white beneath me. That's a "ground blizzard."

We are in the apartment above the clinic this time. Jean chose the "dark" room with its two small and high windows, its own desk, an armchair (with three legs) and a small sofa. I got the gorgeous outer room with only a bed and side table but fantastic view toward East Landing. We are so much farther west that it stays light until almost 8 p.m. (and doesn't get light until 11 a.m.), so I can sit on the bed and feast my eyes. Sometimes it's like one of those glass balls with winter scenes and snow inside. When it swirls heavily I can't even see across the street; then it clears and I can see the boats anchored in the bay. Sometimes the snow packs on the windows and I can't see out at all, until first one piece breaks off, and then another—rather like a jigsaw puzzle.

The apartment is cold, though we each have a small electric-powered radiator in our bedroom. We try to heat the kitchen and bath with the oven. Ice coats the inside of the kitchen windows. The bathroom is fascinating. It has some kind of gas light bulb, I guess, but it is so cold that the gas in the bulb won't ignite. We have devised a showering system where we get into the shower in the dark and the heat of the water warms the bulb so we can dry off in the light. We can't cheat and run the hot water first or we won't have enough to bathe with.

Everyone is up in arms about a patient with known active tuberculosis who decided to take the plane to Anchorage. He refused to wear a mask and threatened suit if they told anyone what he had. What a jerk! People here thought the feds arrested him when he deplaned in Anchorage, but by that time he'd probably spread it around. I doubt he was arrested.

Jean will be here for only five days or so. She works nights pretty much, which is nice for me because I get to practice my cello when she isn't here. Even with a practice mute I like to be careful of disturbing others. I went over to the school and asked if anyone played the piano and might like to get together for a few sessions. I met Pete, a teacher working as janitor. (The school board won't hire two teachers from the same family, and his wife is the principal and teaches special ed.) He plays very well, and we can use the keyboard at the school. Mike Bucey, the music teacher, wants us to play two concerts, one for the first-graders and one for the second grade. It should be fun. Pete and his wife invited me for dinner, and it was wonderful to have a real meal accompanied by people instead of a book propped open. Also present was a "visiting artist," a nice woman from Fairbanks who played guitar and taught composition.

1-28-95

SATURDAY—THE COMFORT and contentment I feel is hard to believe. It's about 4 degrees with gale winds around 35 mph blowing snow. I am still in the frigid apartment above the clinic. The windows are all frosted over (on the inside) even though the portable heater is working well. By wearing wool socks and a down vest, I am comfortable in the kitchen. Jean has gone back to Anchorage so I blocked her bedroom off and stole the heater rather than use the oven to heat the kitchen and bath. I have finished working for the day and am happily having a good vodka and tonic while listening to Dohnanyi's "Serenade in C for String Trio," the Cleveland Quartet playing my beloved music. My big whoop-de-do for my Saturday night off has been a walk to the store and then up to city hall and along the cliff overlooking Bachelor Beach (so named because the "beach masters," the dominant male seals, won't allow the younger males to compete for the females; they drive the youngsters out, leaving them to hang out by themselves on "Bachelor Beach"). So much blowing snow I couldn't see even to the beach. I returned home for the music and drink, then dinner of the frozen caribou meatloaf and butternut squash I brought from home, followed by a Sherlock Holmes tape (VCR) from the library. I had hoped Peter would call to do a little music of our own but the weather is so foul I'm sure no one wants to go out unless they must.

The ice pack bears down upon us and when it gets here the boats will move out, heading for home ports, and the weather is supposed to change. My friends at the clinic promise me brilliant sunshine, cold and clear. But I bet the wind still blows. I can't even see across the road right now, and though Reeve Aleutian Air has canceled flights for today, Security Air is going to try to get in around 7 p.m. I wouldn't bet on it. Reeve is so experienced that when they cancel it usually means the weather is not flyable. Maybe it is with GPS. There is no instrument landing system out here. We have a bunch of patients to send out—back injuries, fractures, head injuries, an amputation with finger to be re-sewn make up the usual fishing mayhem.

Another boat must have arrived with more injuries—I hear much stamping down below in the clinic. If it is the boat that called two hours ago, it is another crush injury of two fingers and amputation of one. What a brutal night. I'm off until noon tomorrow and am old enough not to get involved unless they call me. I will have the duty soon enough.

1-29-95

SUNDAY MORNING AFTER a wonderful night's sleep—Wind blowing as hard as ever but the plane must have gotten in somehow because the beds downstairs in the clinic are now empty. Even the malingerer, who would claim any symptoms in order to go home, is gone, thank goodness. I am treating myself to Mr. Coffee real drip coffee instead of yuck coffee bags this morning. Think I'll have pancakes and one of my precious oranges, then two or three hours of cello practice before I go on call. Cozy, with the wind howling outside. I presume the ice pack isn't here as yet.

· ·

Now I can relate the tale of last night's flight. Today I took care of two passengers from the flight who were coming to work on a processor—I saw them because they had frozen their ears just walking from the plane to the Pribilof expediter's taxi that picked them up. They said they were letting down in zero visibility and the pilot told them he wasn't going to land—just make a pass to show he tried, and head back to Anchorage. The snow drifts so bad here that Dave took four hours to go the five miles to the airport. It was dark, of course, and there wasn't even a quarter-mile visibility. It was a Bering Sea storm!

The passenger who was sitting near the pilot said they suddenly hit a downdraft and dropped 400 feet in an instant, in whiteout. The pilot did what inexperienced pilots do—tried to pull up, which caused a stall that dropped them faster, but somehow was lucky enough to hit the runway, which had to be down there somewhere. He shut it down and got the plane stopped. He couldn't see the runway lights at any time. It's almost unbelievable that they weren't all killed. The visiting artist was to have gone out on that plane but said, "No way!" and happily gave her seat to one of our injured. I would have taken the pilot's name to be sure I never flew with him again in any kind of weather. All of our injured wanted to go with him. I guess if you love risk-taking enough to be a crabber, you love risk-taking enough for anything.

Dave said he had trouble finding the runway from the loading area, and it surely must have been drifted as all else was. When I talked with the Pribilof expediter, who ferries people to and from the airport, she was still goggle-eyed. She said she had watched for a minute as the plane disappeared, and then, as she was on the road at the end of the runway, they passed over her (barely), going the other direction. I hope someone who witnessed it complains to FAA (Federal Aviation Administration). Dave had to lead the caravan back, while breaking drifts. He couldn't see well enough to stay on the road and led them onto the tundra. Fortunately he finally found the road again. The weather is supposed to break about 2 a.m. tonight and in fact already looks better.

Two more patients with ice injuries came in today. One had a 400-pound piece fall from the mast and hit him on the head and back. He is not feeling so good. Told him I thought he was pretty lucky to be here at all. He has a broken shoulder and a lot of bruising. The day has been busy. No cello practice. Dave and I worked from 8 a.m. until about 9 p.m. with a lot of injuries coming in with the boats. There were contusions, lacerations, tendonitis, fractures, dislocations—the whole orthopedic array plus the more mundane aches and pains of the villagers and their families. We had time for lunch by eating a few bites while writing charts. We have another four or five patients to send out tomorrow.

1-31-95

TUESDAY—I CAN'T BELIEVE I had yesterday off but I guess I did. I took the camera down to the dock and got pictures of fishing boats cutting through ice to get to the processors.

Foxes everywhere—couldn't take pictures of boats without them in the foreground. None of the boats was ice-laden, though. I've seen them much worse in Dutch. Pleasant morning and then Pete and I practiced for our performance Thursday. We will do "The Merry Widow Waltz" and "Barcarole." I want to involve the kids so will try to get one from each class to bow on the D string while I finger the notes as I once saw Yo Yo Ma do.

When I came back after practicing the clinic was packed, so I pitched in for a time to help Dave. One poor bad-luck man—when his plane couldn't get in, due to weather, the boat that had hired him left without him so here he is with no money and no job. He was on the docks looking for work. He had swung down onto a deck on a rope and dislocated his shoulder. We relocated it but a man in a sling isn't going to find work. I told him to quit while he was ahead and go home.

This must be what the old frontier and gold rush days were like. It seems to me that there are two kinds out here. The most numerous are the ones I refer to as having dollar signs for eyes. They will do anything for a buck, which frequently enters their nose. The others, whom I love, see the beauty and love the wildness of the weather, the challenges that make them feel alive, and there are some who are really wedded to the sea. When I talk to them after "binding their wounds" I see them come alive, and nothing matters so much as the wondrous life they are leading.

When we finished work, I took a nice long walk. All of Gorbach Bay near Bachelor Beach was clogged with moving ice, a sign of the approaching ice pack. The sea was a lovely greenish white, with beautiful patterns that changed. The surf still pounded on the shore, so the bay was by no means still. I would have stayed for hours, but it was too cold. I walked out on the dunes between town and East Landing. It felt so good after the storm.

Work was really hard today. One unfortunate man's father had just died a few months ago. Then his mother had an auto accident and was in a coma for two weeks. He had decided to come fishing anyway. He had ulcer symptoms and said, "I just shouldn't ever have come," and began to cry. I gave him a medical discharge home.

I took my walk again tonight and the bay looked completely different and not pretty at all. The ice was gone and the color a silty gray. I was astounded after the beauty of yesterday. I wasn't quite to the Point when I heard sirens and saw smoke billowing from one of the village houses. I got back as fast as I could in case we had burn cases or smoke inhalation. It turned out to be Pribilof Expediter's taxi that had burned. Glad no one got hurt.

My homemade humidifier backfired on me. The air in this apartment is so dry that my nose bleeds, so I filled a pie pan with water to put on top of the heater. I felt so smart. I put a second pan on the one in the kitchen. When I got back to the bedroom that pan was already dry and there was a huge wet spot on the rug. Darn thing was leaky as a sieve. Ah well, I left the heater on and the rug was dry again by tonight.

Oh, I forgot to say that when I was walking I looked into the gray infinity and could already see the ice pack. It can't be more than 10 miles off shore. It gives me a strange feeling. Reminds me of how I feel on being snowbound. Nice in a way —makes the pace slower and the priorities different, with a whole new rhythm. The fishing fleet will leave for home, the processors will shut down, all traffic will be by air (when the weather permits), and everyone will depend more on their own supplies because the store will usually be out of many things. (They will come in on the next plane—maybe.) There will be basketball games and fish pie sales to raise money and Bingo, of course. The population will shrink from thousands to about 600, the people who live here year-round—the Natives, the biologists, the Fish and Game people and always, the Coast Guard.

2-3-95

FRIDAY—8 A.M., AND WHAT a night! In fact, the last two days have been fierce. A wave hit while a boat was lifting one of those 7×7×3-foot crab pots—this one full, 700 pounds—and it swung and nailed two men. Fortunately it didn't knock them into the water. The one with the broken shoulder also had a compound fracture of his jaw and I'm sure facial bones as well. Fortunately his eye sockets are OK. Turned out he was from Custer, Washington, 16 miles from where I grew up. The weather is so rotten we haven't been able to get him out.

I'm so tired I guess I'd better go chronologically or I will get lost. The Custer man and his buddy were from my night on call, so I had yesterday off. It was the day of our big school concert—I had gotten only three hours sleep, but the show must go on. We had a ball! I told the kids that "Barcarole" was Italian for *baidarka* (the sealskin boats the Aleuts use), and they thought that was OK. When we swung into the "Merry Widow Waltz" they loved it. All of them, in jeans and sweaters, began waltzing around the room, and I do mean all.

Great fun. Then the two little kids who had practiced bowing did their stuff while I fingered the notes of "London Bridge Is Falling Down." They were so pleased with themselves and got lots of encores. Then the kids brought out recorders and tootled along while Pete and I played one of their songs. Afterward I let them fool around with the cello. All of them were curious. (When my cello was seen as I got in to town, the word went around that I had a big guitar.) I don't think they had seen or heard one before. It was a great success, including the Michigan fight song. Pete and I really enjoyed ourselves.

What made it especially enjoyable was that later, when the high school band heard of our concert, they asked if they could play one for Pete and me! What a once-in-a-lifetime event! Pete and I clapped until our hands were sore. It was especially poignant because there is a very high rate of suicide among the teen-age population here. I weep every time I hear of one leaping off the cliffs. The school is trying to encourage the arts, and the village is trying to include the children in the "old ways," in an attempt to improve the situation. The band we heard plays at non-alcoholic, non-drug dances, and the teens love it, with good cause.

I am not a lifetime cellist but started playing when I was in my fifties. My older sister, Jane, plays violin in the Whatcom County Orchestra in Bellingham, Washington. Her two daughters are both musical. Julia plays viola and has taught orchestra in Juneau. Sarah had been playing cello but was ready to give it up. Because it was a very nice cello, Jane asked if I would like it for my son Ben. I thought that was a good idea and bought it. Ben played it for a couple of years and then decided basketball was more interesting. So there it sat.

I had always liked the sound of a cello. Rather than let this one languish, I began to take lessons. I had met and liked Paul

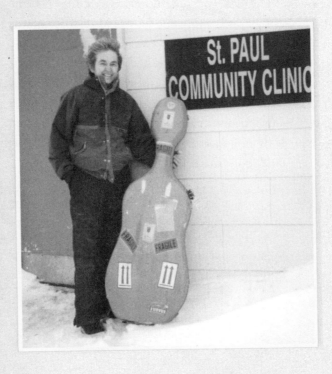

Rosenthal, an excellent musician and director of the Sitka Music Festival. He urged me on, even letting me take a lesson from one of the cellists performing in the festival. I let him know what music I was playing in recitals, once actually had a "musical evening" in my home, and eventually progressed to playing in the Anchorage Civic Orchestra.

Knowing that Paul Rosenthal had a sense of humor, I sent a "newspaper account" of the performance that Peter Schewe and I gave at the school in St. Paul. The famous St. Paul [Minnesota] Chamber Orchestra was of course the inspiration.

St. Paul Chamber Orchestra Scores Big

In a surprise move today the city of St. Paul named Dr. Nancy Sydnam as its principal cellist. Sydnam is well known in Anchorage and Fairbanks for her many dreadful performances and failures before her peers. Especially notable are her timing errors and lamentable intonation.

The initial concerts featuring the works of Lehar and Offenbach were a smash success with the audience, carefully chosen of 1st and 2nd graders who had neither seen nor heard a cello previously. The superb rendition of the "Merry Widow Waltz" had the audience on its feet, living the music.

Equally popular was the familiar "London Bridge is Falling Down." This work, played entirely on the D string, featured members of the audience who assisted Sydnam with the bowing. Multiple encores were called for at both concerts.

A final composition by an unknown Japanese composer, which showcased local recorder artists with cello obbligato, closed the performance.

Dr. Sydnam hopes to make a whirlwind tour with visits to Nikolski and Atka before resuming her duties in St. Paul. The other orchestra member, pianist Peter Schewe, who shone especially brightly in the Michigan victory song, is not pictured.

After supper the day of our school concert a boat called us about a man who, while passing from one boat to another at sea, slipped and fell into the water between the boats. Fortunately there was some sort of fender between the boats that did two things: kept the boats from squishing him and kept him from being blown away on the heavy, frigid seas. Two of his mates saw him fall, jumped into survival suits and leapt into the water with him. By this time he is floating motionless and face down in the ice-filled water. They send a basket down on the crane and haul him up on deck. He is blue as a pair of jeans with no pulse or respiration, but they call us, head for port and give him cardiopulmonary resuscitation (CPR). Darned if he doesn't cough and vomit after about five minutes. It is a first effort at resuscitation for the CPR man, who had just been certified. Not bad. They tried to warm him with hot towels on the way to the dock and I guess they did some good.

But the problem is not over at the dock. There is so much ice in port that they can't get all the way to the dock, so they rig up a ladder catwalk and everyone crawls across it. That ladder ices up pretty fast, too. Dave said the ship swung out and back while he was on the ladder and he wondered if it was long enough. He could feel the ends sliding across the deck. It must have been a real thrill with a 300-pound patient on a stretcher.

By the time the patient got to the clinic, he was barely alive. Core temp of 95 and so blue he looked like one of those blue-faced baboons. Lungs full of fluid, respiratory rate 60, grunting respiration with nasal flaring and a pulse so fast I couldn't count it. Dave is telling me how much better he looks! And he hurts. He is crying with pain. He must feel like his body is one big cramp.

We called a medivac plane from Anchorage. It was a dicey three- to four-hour flight, but the plane made it. We had the grader crew out to clear the road and the runway. I wanted to send the patient with the jaw fracture with them but the grader crew didn't have enough time to extend the available runway to allow for the extra weight. Good evacuation crew from Humana. His O_2 sats (how much oxygen his blood could carry) too low for flying so they tubed him (used an endotracheal tube hooked to a squeezable bag full of oxygen), and I bagged while they got ready to go. We got him up above 90. (Normal is 100%.) When we got him, it was 56 and I thought the machine was broken.

The medivac crew looked like Martians as they left for the airport, with their portable gear on their backs. The weather held and they are on their way to Anchorage. Now I have a whole three hours before I go on call again. Think the commercial flight will get in today. Who knows about tomorrow when I'm to leave for home.

. .

YESTERDAY AFTERNOON ON MY WALK I could see the ice coming in ribbons, streaming in the wind right next to the island. Beautiful and wild. NOW they tell me the weather doesn't get better until the whole island is surrounded by ice.

Range Horse

I heard you in that thick dark before dawn
pawing at the crusty snow beneath my window.
Now I see you, black tail in the wind,
head down, forefoot digging,
your gaunt frame urgent.

Snow frosts your back
as you drift to the church graveyard,
its picket fence open to all that is
and seems to be.

Will old bones nourish yours?
Old dreams keep you whole?

Nikolski

Jan. 15, 1996 — Sunday.

LEFT ANCHORAGE FOR DUTCH HARBOR on Friday the 13th. APIA had chartered Tom Madsen to bring me to Nikolski, but Tom said there were snow squalls and we would try again "tomorrow." My cello arrived in Dutch on its belly, down under a pile of luggage with one catch broken off the case. I phoned for a room at the Grand Aleutian ($110 per night) and stood on the curb to wait for the shuttle. I had waited quite a while when an old patient drove up and asked if I would like a ride to the clinic. Told her no, but I would like one to the hotel. Same old friendly place.

I came out on Reeve—gorgeous for the first $1/3$, then cloud cover with the usual resultant drop to about 1,000 feet over water for miles before the plane got to Dutch. It then skimmed under the lowering clouds at about 500 feet for what seemed forever. Reached Eider Point and made a left turn onto final approach. No wind for a change—rocks and boulders had been blowing across the runway a few days earlier.

It feels good here, and familiar, but the town has changed. There are paved roads with yellow lines! A new hotel, new Carr's grocery (Eagle), new A/C (Alaska Commercial), new post office, new rec center, new footbridge over Town Creek, and new city hall! It is still nice, but different.

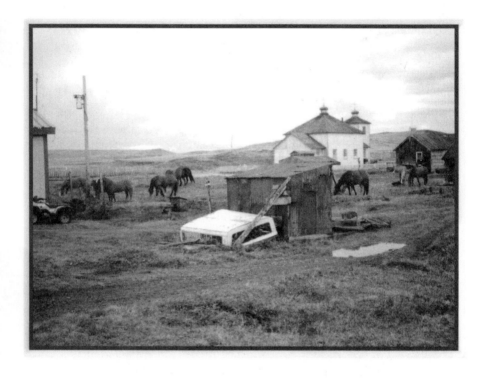

HORSES GRAZE *at* NIKOLSKI, *with the Russian Orthodox
church in the background.*

I packed all my stuff in the room and went for an exploratory walk. I hadn't gotten to my old original duplex when I heard someone shout, "Nancy, is that you?" It was Troy from the clinic—she quit a few months ago. She looks and acts great. She gave me a lift to the clinic where Marlaine was at work. It was so good to see everyone. I walked down to Nicky's Place to see Abi. The store is now complete with an espresso bar and a massage room. She drove me to the dump, where there were more than 200 eagles, then out to her place to see her new computer and to be hugged by her nice black cat, Max. Really. It put its arms around my neck and gave me a big hug. Then she drove us back to town where we had dinner with Marlaine and I got caught up on all the news.

Marlaine came over Sunday morning after breakfast (I had walked to Ziggy's, and there was Bob from the clinic, who insisted on buying my breakfast). Marlaine showed me pictures of her new boat, a 42-foot steel-hulled sailboat named "*Spirit*." It is in Powell River with Axel, her new boyfriend. She and Axel plan to run sailing charters out here with it. That ought to be interesting. She drove us out Captain's Bay Road to see my old emperor geese friends. There must have been hundreds.

I called Tom Madsen, who told me the snow was blowing so hard that we wouldn't even try flying to Nikolski, so I had lunch and took a nap. I got my cooler back from Tom and pulled out a pheasant that I had stuck in frozen on Friday night. It was thawed all right, so I took it along to the "free-for-all" feed at Marlaine's. Bobby and Clare were there, Pete Hendrickson and his black lab, Ebony, and Bob. Dinner was a huge fresh king crab (oh, joy!), sea lion stew (no comment), lamb roast, beans, salad, fresh homemade bread, and blue-berry cobbler over vanilla ice cream. Some good eatin'! Nice people, all. I went home and fell into bed around 11 p.m.

Tom called early today. He was to haul some folks in from Cold Bay at first light and then take me to Nikolski at 1 p.m. Weather looked good for a change. I checked out of the room at noon and watched as the weather deteriorated. By 2 p.m. I didn't think he would make it. Finally at 3 he called and I went tearing out to the airport. He had a nice twin Beech for our journey. We battened cargo and left pronto. He climbed to 700 feet over town and then dropped back down under the fog and snow at Eider Point. Not too bad, though. It finally cleared after we got around that corner. Tom climbed to 2,000 feet and then let me fly. I liked the plane, which cruises at about 140–160 mph. When we got close, Tom took over and buzzed the strip at Nikolski, to be sure there were no cows or horses on it, and came on in. The aide I'm replacing handed me the keys, and the plane left.

1-19-96

FRIDAY—THE BIG DAY! The village kids have been invited to come here to see Wallace and Gromit in *The Wrong Trousers*. I am sure they will love it. I experimented with popcorn last night and found that the big pot makes it perfectly so will have movies, popcorn, and Tang at 3 p.m. I hope they all come.

I am staying at the clinic on a bed in the examining room while Scott and Agrafina Kerr get Lavera Dushkin's house ready to be the new quarters. She has moved to the senior center in Unalaska. I may not move—I'll see. The zone valves here don't work, so there is no heat in the waiting room or the kitchen and all the heat has to filter out from the bedroom and furnace room. There is a wood stove in the waiting room, so that would be a save in cold weather. Only enough wood for about four hours, though.

This is a nice quiet village of about 32 people, and some seem to get up early! I was amazed. There seems to be the usual percentage of alcoholics. Diabetes and hypertension continue to be the worst problems I have seen. Simeon Pletnikoff is charming and interesting. He was a proud member of "Castner's Cutthroats" (also known as Alaska Scouts) and the first man ashore when they retook Attu from the Japanese. Later he showed me his "million-dollar view"—and it is that! His house is near the beach and looks out over the bay with its reef. He has shot sea lion and fur seal from his house. The aide had made him a pot of homemade split pea and ham soup. I had some myself, and was it ever good.

I have tried to walk with Agrafina, but the winds make it hard to go far. We went up North Beach Road one day and put up a flock of huge pintails. Then yesterday we went up "barn way" to the south. A young girl there was breaking a 2-year-old horse to ride. They were having fun. A pond held a flock of teal.

There is no wind right now and I am hoping it stays that way for a few days. I want to explore this weekend. I even brought my compass. Maybe Scott, Agrafina's husband, will take me somewhere or loan me a 3-wheeler. I need exercise!

The mail plane came in yesterday. That poor pilot! I would have ulcers. The weather was rotten, with gusting winds, rain, and poor visibility. He had a huge load of mail and supplies

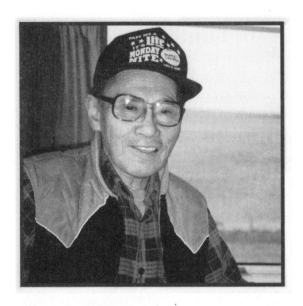

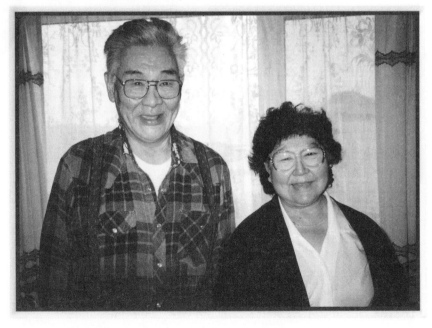

SIMEON PLETNIKOFF, *and* VAL *and* PAULINE DUSHKIN, *all of Nikolski.*

for Chernofski. Because he was taking Art, the ranch manager, from here to there, he came here first. He was to pick up Art and two others but no one told him that Art had 400 pounds of baggage or that the Dushkins were taking a large dog in a kennel. If he had known, he could have (1) taken less gas, or (2) dropped freight in Chernofski on the way down. Art had to leave half his stuff here, including a side of beef. I told Art to say hi to Milt and Cora. The Goose got off the runway in about 200 feet in that wind, but I don't know how the pilot will do on water with that load when he gets to Chernofski with no runway. Pull it up on the beach fast, I guess.

1-20-96

SATURDAY—I'M 67 TODAY, and what does it say on the "inspirational" calendar as I turn to this date? Ah—"Participate." I suppose that is better than yesterday's: "Having lots of money isn't important. Being rich is." Yesterday was gorgeous, with sun and only a little wind. In the morning I walked up to Pauline Dushkin's toward the water tower. Beautiful walk along the bay and then up the hill. Simeon may have the million-dollar view, but Pauline and Val have the two-million-dollar view, just because they are up higher. Pauline showed me the basket she is weaving. She does beautiful work. It is much too tedious for me, although she offered to teach me. If I were to be here for a couple of months I'd take her up on it. She gave me smoked salmon to take home. She uses driftwood for her smoke and this was cottonwood from who knows where. Nice visit.

I was right—the kids all loved Wallace and Gromit. Gabby Danny, nephew of Agrafina and Scott, had seen it before. They went through all my apples, a gallon of Tang and two huge bowls of popcorn. It was a delightful evening. Agrafina borrowed the film last night, so I know it must have gotten rave reviews.

After the kids left I cleaned up and walked north to the now abandoned DEW site. That's along another beach road to the north. Beautiful creeks empty into the bay. I'm sure they are full of salmon in summer.

. .

MY FRIEND BARBARA JUST CALLED TO say "Happy Birthday," so the day is off to a good start even though it looks to be windy and rainy. I borrowed a thermos from Agrafina so I may go trekking to Sandy Beach anyway. I wish I had brought my little gas stove.

Now my birthday breakfast of pancakes, homemade syrup, and eggs is over and I'm treating myself to a second cup of Folger's bag coffee while I decide whether to go out in what did turn out to be wind and rain. Simeon just called to apologize for not showing up for his two-hour postprandial (two hours after eating) blood sugar last night—he says he fell asleep. I set him up again for tomorrow night. We'll see.

I think I'll play my cello for a while. The wind is from the east and it will be all in my face if I go out—well, to the left of my face. Maybe the rain will stop later. I must be getting old to let weather determine my actions. That is OK, too.

1-21-96

SUNDAY—I DID GO for a walk. I packed a lunch and the thermos and set off past the barn to "Sandy Beach." (I think that just means the gravel is less coarse.) The wind wasn't too bad, and it only rained part of the time. Not a single glass ball! I walked all the way down to South Point, or what I thought was South Point. Found what looked like a float cemetery— so many of them, but none glass. Beautiful reefs, harlequin ducks, surf against the gravel that makes that lovely tinkling sound on the outward phase. My beloved emperor geese were on the rocks at the point. I really wanted to get a picture there but they were too spooky. Some small reddish ducks got out of the tide pool as I turned the corner.

It took about three hours to get there but only two and a half to get back. The wind picked up and I couldn't find a good spot for lunch. I finally found a niche in the cliff this side of Sandy Beach, full of colorful lichens and out of the wind. I played tag with the emperors all the way, then climbed the cliff right after lunch and came home north of the water tower across the fields on a 4-wheeler track. It felt good to be physically tired.

· ·

AFTER DINNER MY GRANDSON STORM called. Hearing his voice was a pleasure. His birthday is the same as mine. I will never forget it for several reasons. My lovely, rebellious daughter, Claire, was living in Kotzebue when she got pregnant. "Wonderful," I said. "You can come home six weeks prior to your due date and one of our obstetricians can deliver you here in our hospital." Of course she wouldn't have it that way. She had already made plans to see an Eskimo midwife during the pregnancy and then have a home delivery. No amount of wailing about the dangers of a first baby delivered at home made any difference, even after I sent her a bumper sticker that read "Home Deliveries Are for Pizzas." Stubborn child! Then when she was fairly near term the midwife quit her practice to have cataract surgery. Claire and I formed a new pact stating that she would fly to Anchorage just two weeks prior to her due date. Somehow there was always a reason she couldn't come in.

I was at work in my office the morning she called to tell me she was in labor. I knew all the flight schedules by heart so happily told her that was great and she would just have time to make the flight to Anchorage. "Mom, I'm not going anywhere," she said. She says I hung up on her, and I probably did. I canceled my office schedule and tore to the airport to catch the flight to Kotzebue. That plane got in and out of Kotzebue just before a tremendous storm hit—the worst one in 50 years, with heavy snow and high winds. Claire labored through the afternoon, and when it got to be time to go to the hospital her house was snowed in with eight-foot drifts surrounding it. Ever creative as one must be in the Bush, the village leaders sent a front-end loader to pick her up. The driver extended the shovel over the snowbank, and between her contractions she climbed into the bucket to be transported to the other side where a police car waited to take her to the hospital. There was no room for me in the car and the wind was so strong that I couldn't even stand up, so I had to crawl most of the way to the hospital. Ropes were strung up along the roads to keep people from wandering out on the ice and getting lost. It was impossible to see more than a few feet in that ground blizzard.

When the doctors there found out I was a doctor they asked if I would like to deliver her. I told them they had better ask her and was surprised and delighted when she said yes. They quickly got "privileges" for me, an easy task because I had so many years of experience. The delivery went well, with no complications. What deep joy to hand my new grandson to the waiting arms of my daughter. Thus "Storm" and I share our birthdays

He told me about his birthday party, which sounded like fun, and Claire called from work. I certainly don't feel forgotten.

. .

TODAY I SEE fresh snow on the hills, and although it is windy with low-lying stratus, the sky is blue. I have had a shower and washed my hair plus put on a clean shirt so am ready for the day. Scott and Agrafina go to Dutch tomorrow; maybe I'll see if they'll loan me a 3-wheeler and tell me where the hot springs are. West wind today, and when I open the windows I can clearly hear the surf on the beach. Lots of rosy finches at the feeder.

Claire's Ulu

Years ago my son Elliott had a set-net site across Cook Inlet at Granite Point. I would often fly over to visit and pick berries. My sister Ann came with me one day, and I have a picture somewhere of her cavorting in the artesian spring.

One of my best memories of Granite Point is when I flew Claire over. We got lots of salmon that day, and Elliott and Claire had a contest to see who was fastest at cleaning and filleting the fish. Claire with her ulu won hands down over Elliott with his fish knife. They were both just a blur while I cheered them on. We fished for trout and salmon in a nearby stream, and Tigger thought he had to retrieve anything that splashed.

Perfect Day

Beneath green leaves, blue berries cling.
Huge clusters bend the branches down
to kiss the ground from which they spring.
They're hiding so they won't be found,
but we are super sleuths today--
these pails we have aren't just display.

The sun drips heat, no moving air,
ideal for bugs that bite and chew.
They hold town meetings in your hair,
decide who gets which part of you.
The nets, the spray—what's that to them?
For our defense we must use Zen.

The berries mount to fill our pails,
their plump round blueness, globe on globe.
Bug guardians of the berries failed—
we foiled them with the strength of Job.
We're hot with dust, no time to bask
for now we face the final task—

the long walk home, the sun's hot glare.
Then just beyond the second bend
we see it spurting in the air—
artesian well, the traveler's friend.
We cache our pails and run to play
within wet coolness, perfect day.

LATER THAT NIGHT [1-21-96]—THE SUN CAME OUT and the day was beautiful and clear—an occasional snow squall but not much. I found out I had taken a wrong turn at Coast Guard Gate and gone onto the beach instead of keeping high on the tundra, so I didn't ever get to Sandy Beach but only to Camel Rock. Agrafina took me overland on the 4-wheeler. I don't know why speed was important but we literally flew. The pounding probably made me an inch shorter than I was when we started. Pauline, whose house we roared past, called laughing when I got home and advised a long hot tub.

Sandy Beach is indeed sandy—and miles long, with gorgeous surf. I would dearly love to have stayed a while but it was not to be. We tore back to town and took the road out toward Okee Point north of town. As we flew through the air I did see the base of the volcano. I would love to see it on a really clear day.

Suddenly my time here seems too short. Maybe I will try the trail west from the airport to the Pacific side after work.

1-22-96

MONDAY—A BEAUTIFUL clear day—cold in the night with a skiff of snow on the ground this morning. As it got light I could hardly believe my eyes: There was Mt. Vsevidof to the right of the old DEW site, completely white and very majestic. I ran out with my camera and then decided to check on Simeon, whom I'd started on insulin. At his place I looked out the window and could see the Islands of the Four Mountains, across Samalga Pass—Kagamil, Chuginadak with Mt. Cleveland, Carlisle, Yunaska and Amukta. There wasn't even any wind. What a treat!

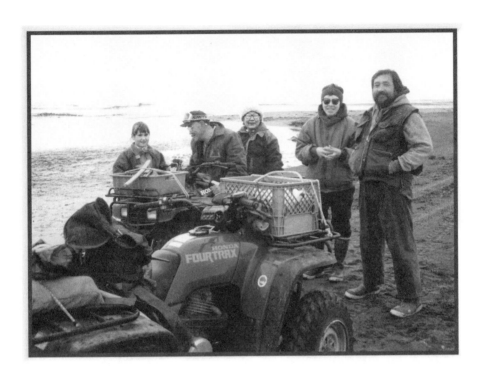

At Nikolski *(from right):* Peat Galaktionoff, Agrafina Kerr, Pauline *and* Val Dushkin, Tatiana Barraclough.

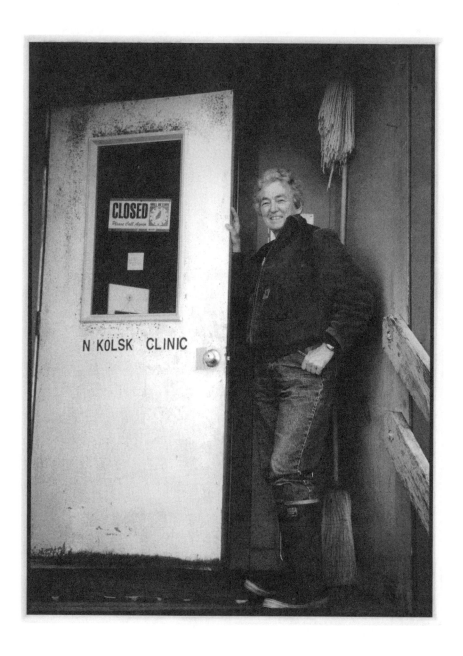

Closing time *at the Nikolski clinic.*

The mail plane got in and Scott, Agrafina and Danny left. I think Peat Galaktionoff was feeling lonely. He and Scott lately paddled their baidarkas to spend two months at the Islands of the Four Mountains (I think of them as the Islands of the Four Volcanoes, although there are five). Anyway, he offered to take me exploring. Days like this are rare indeed, and I took him up on it. We went to the top of the DEW site where there was a breathtaking view of Vsevidof and the jagged mountain next to it. Peat guided Japanese mountain climbers there awhile back. Great view of Anangula Island and the bay, too. The Islands of the Four Mountains were already being covered by clouds so we came down and headed out to "Pacific side," past the lake and east of Sandy Beach, where there's a huge midden. Nice beach, complete with fox who watched us for a while. Whale bones scattered here and there—perhaps they were used to support the roofs of the barabaras. I saw a duck blind at the lake and one formed of logs on the beach, as well as lots of waterfowl. A huge flock of pintails. This was an easier trip than the one with Agrafina.

I came home, had tea, and browsed some books I borrowed from Peat. He is a Native artist who used to teach in Dutch. He knows Ray Hudson, artist and author, there, and Abi, of course. He bartends to make money and then comes out here to live. He seems a very nice young man and is easy to be with. We had planned another adventure tomorrow but I think our good weather has deserted us. The wind is howling and the house shaking. I managed to get a load of washing done at Lavera's house this afternoon, though, so I feel comfortable.

Another big box of supplies came—I must inventory it and get it put away. Seems like a lot of stuff for so few people. I will call Bill Ermeloff back in to recheck his blood pressure and blood glucose. Also have to reach one more woman I wanted to see. I hope it is a good sleeping night.

1-23-96

Tuesday—It wasn't. A real storm has hit. This little old house shakes so bad there are whitecaps in the toilet! The satellite dish must have blown askew—no TV this morning. I am sure I don't want to 4-wheel to South End today—a 2½ hour 4-wheeler ride. On to the box of meds.

Pauline and Val Dushkin made it in for blood checks and blood pressure. I do enjoy them. I got the TV set working again, found a fax message that had been sitting there since the 19th, and discovered the hiding place of the slides for the HemoCue. Bill Ermeloff reported his blood sugars by phone but will not come in until the weather improves.

My bird feeder on the north window has become a bird bath. The water is pouring down both the north and south windows—now it is rain mixed with snow. I imagine the old Aleuts snuggled down inside their barabaras on a day like this. I got to see some barabaras in Point Lay one time when we went up along the coast for a whaling feast. Claire had been invited to be on the cooking crew, which was a great honor, so Ben and I went up. Barabaras are dug into the tundra so that most of the building is underground, and then sod is piled around the edges and over the top. Whale ribs were frequently used to support the roof. Entrance is or was by ladder. The wind doesn't shake a barabara, but just flows over the top. Those Aleuts knew what they were doing.

Strange that I haven't seen any birds flying here.

1-24-96

WEDNESDAY—CALM—no wind! But fog is already rising. I have checked my two diabetics. Peat is offering tea and alodick, a Russian fried bread. I am to invite Simeon as well, after which we will 4-wheel to Driftwood Bay on the Pacific side. I should have opted for the return home next week so I would have the weekend in Nikolski! But then I thought I would have the first one. Planning doesn't do much good out here.

. .

IT IS NOW WEDNESDAY NIGHT—SIMEON in a snit when I got there. His heat had gone out in the night and he was having trouble fixing it. He had not had his insulin. He said he ought to just shoot himself and be done with it. I finally talked him into coming to Peat's with me. The bread was fantastic! I made a real pig of myself—much to Peat's delight. Simeon went home happy, and Peat and I left for Driftwood Bay.

Duck paradise on the way, and just as we arrived there were my emperor geese on shore. Great surf decorated a beautiful bay. A nutty "surfer of the world" is staying in the line shack there and taking pictures for some surf magazine. He was out in the bay in his wetsuit while we were there so I didn't get to meet him. Peat says that when he came into the Elbow Room no one would sit with him because he was so crazy. Now that *is* crazy!

Aleutian Mummies

Learning that the Aleuts of the eastern islands made mummies impressed me greatly. It is difficult to make a lasting mummy! Aleuts are equal to challenges, however. If they wanted to keep the spiritual power of the deceased person around, they would find a way to do that. They didn't need a college course in comparative anatomy for the task – they had sea otters to show them the way. Remembering the long year it took us to dissect a cadaver in medical school, I was surprised to read that the Aleuts also did autopsies. We didn't have years of dissecting sea otters to guide us, however.

I learned from William S. Laughlin's *Aleuts: Survivors of the Bering Sea Land Bridge* that what the Aleuts did was eviscerate the body through an abdominal incision and then stuff it with beach grasses. The next step, after dressing it in its best clothes, was to flex the body, knees to chest, and insert it, along with beads, hunting equipment, baskets and other things of value used by the deceased, into a sort of cradle. This cradle was then wrapped in a woven grass mat and suspended from the ceiling of the barabara – the customary semi-underground dwelling – where the smoke from cooking fires rose and preserved the body. There it remained for months, close to the people who mourned the deceased.

Some barabaras were more than a hundred feet long and shared by multiple families. No one had to walk to a cemetery to visit a loved one. They had only to look to the ceiling to feel closeness again. When the time seemed right to the mourners, the cradle was moved to a nearby cave where it would remain dry.

Lots of good boards for Peat but no glass balls for me. Two dogs appeared from town. Two seals eyed us for a while. I heard stories of Dolly Varden trout hiding in the places where the stream goes underground. Old-timers would block both entrances, then dig a hole and pick them out by hand. They used to dry the peat moss and burn it, too. I told Peat they still do that in Ireland.

There was another midden near the line shack. Must be one on every beach. The largest are at Sandy Beach. They tell me there are many mummies at South End, where I didn't get to go.

. .

I HAVE MY GEAR PACKED, BOOKS READY to return to Peat, charts finished, and wrote a note to the new woman. Now watch—the wind will rise and I will be here for another week. OK by me!

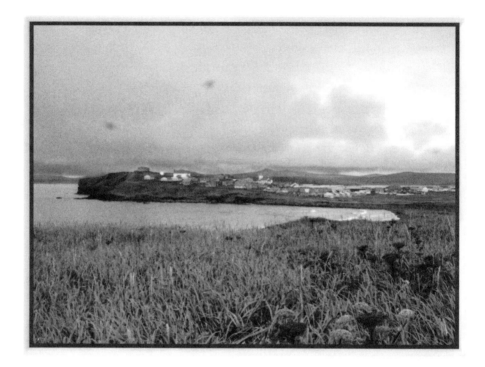

ST. PAUL, *from the other side of Bachelor Beach.*

Tranquility

Unhurried at last, I lie listening
to the hymnal of the world about me.

Each clef with its own song—
basses, treble, tenor
joining, parting,
joining again

while within the melodic whole,
the razor-toothed shark
slides its sleek body, etching
its lines of curves and glissandos,
this time declining explosion into view.

Letters to fellow poetry class students

St. Paul, Nov. 5, 1998 — Thursday.

I hope you all think of me out on this island in the middle of the Bering Sea—and if you do, please remember to speak clearly and distinctly—maybe a little slower than usual so that I may hear what you are saying via the recorder. I can't bear to miss two whole classes. I can turn in the work but that doesn't cut it. It's the wonderful discussions that teach so much. We are learning what works and what doesn't and why. I'm also going to try to have your poems and journals faxed out so I won't get so far behind.

St. Paul is a wonderful place for poets. I guess every place is that, but St. Paul seems particularly so. It is very like Ireland. The first time I came back with pictures, my friends asked what my Ireland photographs were doing in with the Pribilof ones. That's probably not true of November, when it is definitely not green in the Pribilofs. It is still beautiful, though, with the mist-enshrouded beaches deserted and stretching for miles, the blue foxes that come into town in whole clans at night, the young orcas, clearly visible through the blue-green water from my vantage point on a near cliff. I won't suffer too much.

I've been reading about poetry critic Helen Vendler. I love it when she says just what Linda says—"Most poetry has power over us by what it says, not with theme, but with the language in which it enacts the theme. A poem is not an essay. It does not have a topic sentence which it then develops. It is more like a piece of music. It is a constantly evolving form taking new shapes as it goes along." She believes that poetry is meant as much to be heard as it is to be read—sound familiar? She wrote poems as a student but found the results disappointing. She says they were the poetry of statement rather than waywardness—they came from thought rather than imagination and were therefore expository. And doesn't that sound familiar, too? I worry that my line, like hers, is analytical rather than imaginative. Reading Robert Hass makes me worry even more because I'm so restricted that I have difficulty following him. The only comfort is that I'm not static, I'm looser than I used to be.

St. Paul, Nov. 12, 1998—Thursday.

No Oscar nominee could possibly have waited with more anticipation than I for the arrival of the poetry class envelope. There was a 22-foot ceiling that day with 50-knot crosswinds on the one runway. Good old Reeve made it in anyway. Oh, joy, oh, bliss! I didn't get it until 10 p.m. but stayed up until 1 a.m. listening and then reading all the journals. Thanks to you all for your efforts!

I see from Linda's handouts that the one Hass book the library didn't have is the one I should have gotten. I feel as though I've entered a foreign country and don't know the language. I'm not even sure my passport is valid. This is all so contrary to my linear-thinking, analytical medical training.

I read and reread and by the third time begin to get the gist. I'll slit my throat if the rest of you just breeze through saying, "Oh, yeah." (Two beats.) Anyone else find him abstruse?

Some of his concepts are fascinating. Taking the pleasure derived from recognition of form back to the pleasure an infant feels in the pattern of hunger, food, affection, and pleasure, which we all experience, is one I like.

The one about form being the skeleton the reader can use to constellate her imaginings is less clear to me. It must be like the constellation of archetypes, which I barely understand. I think I need to go to a cave with no distractions for a while.

Tonight's distraction was a seal bite. This poor guy was rigging his crab pots in the dark and walked to the water's edge to pee. What he thought was a rock to walk on was a seal that was probably sound asleep. What a gash— right down to the bone. Now, I can tell you about the layers, which bone, which sutures to use on fascia, which for skin, and it is easy and straightforward. I don't have to concern myself with his personal resolution of the opposite pulls of merging and separation. Or do I? He had been drinking heavily. (Read: He has feelings with which he either doesn't want or is unable to deal.) Crabbing is a very dangerous, "far out" occupation. Maybe he misses his wife back home. Maybe it makes him feel closer to his mother for us to care for him. Suddenly this nice straightforward thing that I am so sure I know all about—one with a clear-cut beginning and ending—is a thick soup of possibilities. I guess I will take the soup every time, because it's a whole person who got bitten, not just a leg. And I suppose that is why I like this class so much. It is frustrating because the answers aren't a clear-cut formula, but, oh, the richness of the soup. This ain't no see-through broth, gang.

St. Paul, Nov. 19, 1998 — Thursday.

It took three trips to the airport to get the envelope this week, but it came. Judith need not have rushed. The plane went to Dillingham but couldn't get in out here so returned to Anchorage and then tried again in the late afternoon. Success! I roared back to my quarters, where the heat had gone off as it mysteriously does. Fixed a vodka and tonic, turned the electric heater on, tucked my cold toes under, and leaned over it with a floppy shirt so the heat rose and warmed me while I read.

I wrote the pantoum I did this week because I get so upset about what seems like an epidemic of mental illness in this village. The last time I was here, four teenagers in separate incidents had jumped off the cliffs to die. It's like moving mountains to get changes made. I asked about it this trip and learned that one girl had jumped this year. I suppose one is better than four, but there shouldn't be any. I guess this isn't the place to discuss social problems, but I see more here than seals and beaches.

On to poetry—Why does anyone want to change the name of Marissa's poem? I love both the poem and the title. I think it is perfect with her revision. It has been almost 50 years since I saw my first Van Gogh and it is just as she says:

I still remember it vividly and in detail. Stunning is much too small a word. Like Marissa, I felt captivated and drawn in. If she feels that way about someone, look out, world!

Maybe I haven't been clear. I don't think using the title of the picture she saw is appropriate because it doesn't make any difference which picture. The point is that she had never seen his work before and when she did—Smackeroo! And there can only be one first time. She might go back and see the same canvas or different ones and be moved by them, but it will never have the same impact, that heart-stopping wonderment. No catalogue or reproduction conveys an iota of what the original does. I think it is a good and joyful thing to lust after someone you know you can never have. To me it seems a part of living life with vigor and passion. Reach, reach, reach, that's what we are all doing in this class.

Now it is Sunday night and I have lapsed into coma. The heating system, which has been off for two days, has become repentant and in atonement is supplying two days' heat in one or two hours. The only movable window is on the windward side, and when I open it a crack the wind drives the rain in, soaking the rug. What really bugs me is that I have trouble hearing Dvorak over the wind, the groaning of the quarters, and the various rattlings.

I have finally figured out Robert Hass. I think the man is certifiably crazy. Some of what he writes is classical schizophrenic flight of ideas. He is so brilliant that he uses meter and rhythm to hold it, and probably himself, all together. His "beasts" are really beasts. He disassociates to a marked degree. It is fascinating to me how if I read what he writes without trying to understand the words, the clauses, the rambling sentences—if I just go on aloud I almost know what he means. I don't think I'm able to go as far afield as he is, but I'd be willing to bet that he occasionally needs help getting back. Then in the midst of a lot of goop will come a gorgeous phrase like "Longing, we say, because desire is full of endless distances" (hear that, Marissa?), and I just want to melt, knowing he is so right. Strange man.

Enough, must get packed in case the plane makes it in tomorrow. Hope I get to join you and pass these out in person.

St. Paul, March 24, 1999 — Wednesday.

While Bill and Susan had a wonderful week with actual sleep time, my spring break has been just the opposite—18-hour days in St. Paul during the crabbing season. It is cold here, so I do my reading in bed. The lamp sits atop Carruth, Gwynn, Oliver, and Wallace, stacked on my class notebook on top of a food cooler—my nightstand. I was hoping I'd have time to work ahead and at least start a villanelle but it's been so hectic that I haven't even got decent ghazals. What little time I have is interrupted. With 35-foot seas those boats just won't hold still, which means the clinic is busy. Worse is when whole boats go missing, as one did this morning. Even in survival suits they can't be alive by this time.

And now it is Saturday a.m. The plane that was to take me home got in yesterday, but somehow they canceled my reservation and the flight was full. Kent, my replacement, and I stopped at the Coast Guard station to ease our pain with a couple of Coronas. He is a young pig farmer from Delta and had loaned me his book of Robert Frost's poems while he went home for a week. It is very well-worn, with some pages falling out. It pleases me that he has it, he loves it, and he wants to share it. The introduction is written by Louis Untermeyer, who says that Frost waited 20 years from writing his first poem to publish his first book. At first I was daunted—do I have 20 years to get command of the art? And then I realized that he published what he had been writing during those 20 years. Untermeyer quotes a critic on Frost's poems praising "their rich enjoyment of all kinds of practical life." That is what I would like to be able to do. I have had this incredibly rich, enjoyable life and something in me wants to set it down on paper. Did I wear wool to catch the cockleburs? We will see.

At least I feel better about my literary taste. I read Carruth on Frost. (I enjoy Carruth no end and that in itself is a sign of good taste.) In his essay he compares "Stopping by Woods on a Snowy Evening" with "For Once, Then Something." I had the preconceived notion that "real poets"—published ones—never published poems that weren't wonderful. I know, I know—Linda has been trying to tell us that isn't so, but it seems to take a while to de-solidify my thoughts. When I read "For Once . . ." I didn't like it; without reading on, I tried to write down my reasons for not liking it. I didn't get all that Carruth did but it was close enough, so I charged on to "Two Tramps in Mud Time," using Kent's book. Here Carruth talks of four stanzas of editorializing. Since that is a concept I seem to have difficulty understanding, I really studied those four stanzas. It seems to be ego insertion, judgment, conclusions. He didn't tell by showing, he told. What a slippery art this is.

The whole point of the essay was that Frost, with his wonderful craftsmanship, forced many of his poems instead of allowing them to be "open to experience—and not only open but submissive, and not only to experience, but to the actual newness of experience here and now." In other words, be sure you have your lights on and that you wear wool to catch the cockleburs.

That is my literary discovery. My practical discovery is that in this building erected in the 1920s, when the wind blows from the northwest—the side the vents are on—none of the toilets will flush; in fact, they will overflow. Guess where the wind is coming from this morning.

Nancy

Lost Between Crab and Cod

There is something appealing about this storm,
the comfortable lostness of it.
The school across the street
has ceased to exist.
The cemetery on the hill,
store on the corner, post office,
airstrip down the road, all
are gone and the village hangs suspended

between seasons of crab and cod,
breathes easily in this storm,
the familiarity of snow hung
softly about its shoulders,
snow that could smother but says: Rest—

stay in the warmth of family.
Speak sweet words in gentle Native tongue.
Bake fish pie in leisure, you've nowhere to go.
No need to hide the longing look.
Let it linger between you
while the storm blusters on.

No loved ones ride waves
from crest to crest,
the suck and release of
the downward plunge
hypnotic in its horror as the
rigging ices up.
Not this time—
You're between crab and cod.
Let your selves be lost.

St. Paul

June 7, 1999 — Monday.

IT IS MY KIND OF SUNDAY MORNING — public radio from Juneau playing classical music, rainy and foggy out — I can barely see East Landing — and all the villagers still in bed. And most important, I slept all night for the first time since I have been here. Feel like my old self instead of the wreck I have been since the start of this trip. Like a fool, I neglected to bring my music tapes — a big mistake I will not make again.

Stalwart Pauline Rukovishnikoff, one of the best village aides, is gone this trip but I've gotten to know Jama, another aide, who is helpful and a lot farther along than I recall. We got a gastrointestinal bleeder in a little after midnight, and Jama was excellent. She threaded the IV's in while I pushed the Zantac. His hemoglobin was only 6.8 gm (normal is 12–14 gm.). Of course, the weather was thick with fog so we couldn't medivac him out. Shades of my first tour here.

I will never forget that "first time" in St. Paul. I had another GI bleeder who had come to make his fortune fishing. As ever, the weather prevented medivac from getting in so I sat with him through the night in that little back room. We talked as his life ebbed. "Gee," he said," I always wanted to see the village of St. Paul, and here I am but I can't see it." To myself I said, "If you see the sun rise you will be lucky." Strange the effect of being close to someone so near the precipice that decides between life and death. I held his hand a long time while taking his pulse, the puny IV drip doing its best. He turned out to be lucky. He made it. But it was sure close.

Now with this bleeder, the medivac crew promised us to be here by noon or 1 p.m., and we held our breath as his hemoglobin dropped to 4.8. I socked him with 150 mg of Zantac in one bolus, which at least slowed him enough so he had tarry stools instead of straight un-clotted blood. The medivac team got as far as King Salmon and then weather forced them to go back to Anchorage. They promised to be back here by 5:30 p.m. Hemoglobin dropped to 4—no plane—refueling—7:30 p.m., hemoglobin 3.8. They finally got here with one lone unit of O negative blood. I am sure it helped. He wasn't in shock and was nice and warm, with a strong, regular pulse at 70, but I knew he would crash when they moved him. They had pressure bags around his IV's before they left and I'm sure they used them. I called two days later and he was still in intensive care. They had done a vagotomy, taken his gall bladder out, were still giving him blood, and had him almost up to 8 gm. I feel pretty good that we kept him alive.

· ·

TIME FOR BREAKFAST. I HAVE EGGS TO DEVIL if it clears enough for a hike. I want to go overland out the NW road. Yet another holiday tomorrow—Aleut Day, with a big barbecue at the school plus music and dancing. Should be fun.

6-9-99

WEDNESDAY—I HAD planned a walk after work today but at 4:15 p.m. we got a 34-year-old with a heart attack (acute myocardial infarction). He was scared out of his wits and I wasn't far behind, but medical management really hasn't changed all that much. The basics are still the same. I wasn't sure about the beta blockers, but the rest was just like old times. Becky Abbott Lundquist's medivac training manual is a perfect jewel of clarity! A 6-year-old who could read could follow it. The patient did well once I managed his pain. He had stable blood pressure and pulse and was never in respiratory distress. The aide and I were glad when the plane got in because the weather was dicey as usual. I feel really good about how well both our tough cases have gone. Medicine is still fun and I still do an adequate job.

I did go out to Tsammanah and Lincoln Bight on Sunday afternoon. Weather was gorgeous—sunny, mild wind. Foxes walked with me along the high bluffs north of SW Point, and there were lots of birds. Sat and ate lunch with a fox watching me. Not another soul around. I felt content and at peace and a part of all that surrounded me—the same harmony I hear in music, all the different notes making a beautiful song. Near the bight I met two Fish and Feathers (Fish and Game agents) who nearly fainted to see another human way out there. They were on 4-wheelers making bird counts along the high bluffs. They said the best birdwatching was from the beach and I could walk it the entire way. I looked and it was all boulders and I knew it would have been rough going. I stuck to the high ground. Great beachcombing at Lincoln Bight. Ann would have found a glass ball, I'm sure. A good hike. Jama, who lives here, has never been out there. Too bad.

My next goal is to drive out past the airport, Lake Hill and Little Polovina, then park and hike to Marunich. I bet the beachcombing is good there. I got almost there from West Rookery along the sands, the first Sunday I was here, but my head was such a mess at the time that it wasn't much fun. Hard with Mother's death in January, and now Claire, my daughter, is very ill with pulmonary sarcoid that seems unresponsive to anything. I try to focus on just what is here today and seem to have settled in OK. I think it helps enormously to be busy, and to be successful on a couple of dire cases.

Aleut Day was great. I made a Waldorf salad complete with cherries. They had three or four grills going, with reindeer sausage, hamburgers, hot dogs, and FRESH CRAB! It was very good. Then their dance group did Aleut dances. The kids were about junior high age, I think, and were wearing beautiful full-length sealskin dresses made by the elders in the elder home here. I have never seen anything like them. The faces of the children are even more beautiful. I chatted with their director and told her how nice it was, and enjoyed talking with people a little. I was surprised at how many I knew. I met a new Fish and Feathers volunteer from Whidbey Island in Washington state. She seemed a nice girl. I miss Pauline Rukovishnikoff. I know she would have been there if she were in town.

Well, I've calmed down enough to sleep, I hope. Last night was the pits. I hope I get my walk tomorrow. Tom put air in the low tire on the 4-wheeler—relief.

᷈

*I*N AUGUST OF 1999, MY DAUGHTER, CLAIRE, became increasingly ill with pulmonary sarcoid. This is often a terminal disease, and while my lifetime of medical knowledge and experience could not help her, it was sufficient to terrify me. The leading expert in the disease was in Seattle, so Claire, her now-ever-present oxygen tank and I flew there. Friends Margaret and Bill Sharrow recognized my coping limits and presented us with first-class upgrades. Their generosity made the trip much more comfortable for Claire and therefore easier for me.

Claire was immediately admitted to the University of Washington hospital for lung surgery. Sadly, the damage was worse than anticipated. Although she fought very hard to stay alive, she lost that battle 10 days after surgery. She left not only her three brothers, her dad, and me, but two sons: Storm, age 17, and Cornelius, 8.

When her house in Wasilla was sold I set up a trust fund for the two boys, to cover their future needs. Storm started college and my son Ben and his wife moved to Anchorage from Portland to care for Cornelius.

Letter from Adak

Adak, AK, Nov. 18, 1999

Dear Ann,

I feel rather like Alice having dropped down the rabbit hole. I am alone in this huge deserted building (Navy hospital). All the clocks read a different time, which adds to the surrealistic effect, the wind & rain pound outside & it's cold as hell in here. I have little heaters on in the 3 rooms I intend to use. The PA left today on the plane. That would have been OK, but Denise, on whom the entire operation depends, left as well since her grandfather just died. She of the keys and maps of this old dinosaur, she who answers the phone, makes appointments, shows me where to find things. I pray there is no real emergency. Takes me 15 minutes to find a tongue depressor.

My first appointment today is for a hepatitis B shot. The patient is now 5 minutes late, but after diligent searching I have found the vaccine & the syringe & needles. No luck so far with the chart. Do have the chart of the guy from yesterday. Someone smacked him across the nose with a 2×4. Ken had seen him & sewed him up & packed his broken nose. Called me to see him yesterday since he had a bone fragment protruding from his septum. It costs $1,100 round trip to Anchorage, so we decided we'd try to remove it. Ken couldn't, but old Cool Hand Luke (me) could. He was a great patient. Then we stuffed his periostium back under the mucosa & sent him home. Told him he owed me $1,100.

Since we had the unprecedented luxury of two practitioners at once, Ken took Tuesday off (a SUNNY day) & I had yesterday off (pouring rain, wind & hail). We each had a car—me a huge long-bed Ford 350LR 4×4, he a cute little Bronco (now mine). I drove out to Clam Lagoon, which is alive with otter. Lots of harlequin ducks as well. Came back for lunch & worked on the nose & then drove to Finger Inlet & hiked up to Belly Lake. The lake is ugly but the climb up along the stream with its multiple waterfalls was spectacular. A few caribou tracks but that was all. The weather so foul I didn't feel like sitting & glassing the area. Took quite a few pictures, one of the base housing with the things that look like air conditioners at the windows. It's actually a protective shield so you can open the window without having the rain come in.

This is clearly a U.S. Navy base & has none of the ambience of a Native village. It is palpably different. The cafeteria where we all eat is in the high school, as is the gym, weight room, sauna & full size swimming pool. Also administrative offices. Our quarters are very nice—new & clean, lovely furniture. I wish I'd brought my own food as the cafeteria is very so-so & the kitchens in quarters very well equipped.

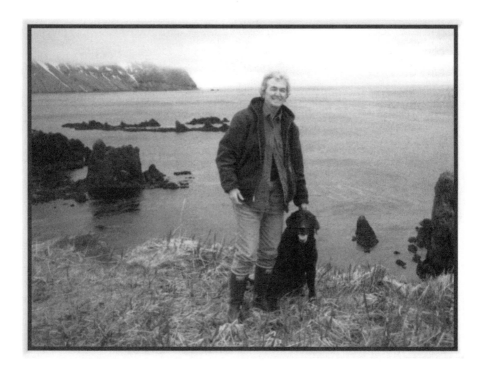

With Tigger *at Adak.*

It would be wonderful to have a boat here. Boyd was here with the Navy & had a wonderful time. He will think me very tame to have explored in a truck. I have seen some islands through the mist once in a while—the ones to the east.

Have already read half my book supply—we rented *Horse Whisperer* last night (don't bother). Think I'll get another tonight. I work until 8 tonight, not having started until noon. That's because the indispensable Denise works also for Reeve & the flight gets in at 11:30 or 12 on Monday & Thursday, therefore clinic doesn't start on those days until noon.

APIA called yesterday & asked me to work in Nikolski December 2 through 9. If I get out of here on time & get to go to Victoria I'll probably do it. The $$ are welcome & I will have spent time with Cornie. Want to come? Let me know so I can clear it with Harriet. We go out on mail plane after overnight in Dutch @ hotel. You'll probably be getting ready for Egypt.

Well, my hepatitis shot hasn't shown so I will huddle closer to the heater & read.

Did I tell you that when I went to the bank to get the balance of the boys' trust account (they only send paper quarterly), she gave me a figure that was way too high. I told her she had the wrong account, but she showed me a deposit I didn't have. Little Valley Hospital, where Claire worked (and Cornie was born), has donated over $18,000. I nearly fainted and began to cry. What do you say to people like that? Don't you begin to get a different picture of Claire from that old rebellious destructive teenager? I wanted to go talk to the administrator but came out here so haven't.

And now everyone has come at once—the fire chief with parameters for "respiration tests." Someone else with a batch of tests to be run. The hep B shot & a tennis elbow and someone wanting info faxed RIGHT NOW. Ah, Denise, you are without price!

Had a great time with Carol O. I'm so lucky to have such wonderful friends. Will try to call you on the WATS line this weekend.

Love,
Nancy

. .

POSTSCRIPT: I had one other monthlong trip to Adak, in May 2000, on which I got permission to bring my lab, Tigger, for company. That wasn't easy because the Navy was still the boss on the island and prohibited non-sterilized dogs from admittance. They finally let me bring him after I pointed out that if the other dogs had been fixed, there wasn't much danger from him.

What a difference it made having him there with me. It was so nice to have someone waiting at home. We took long walks on the beaches and in the hills. I also met Phyllis Walters, an NP (nurse practitioner) who worked with me. She loved to hike as much as I did and showed me lots of her favorite places.

Artist in Waiting

For Cornelius

There he goes. Straight as a horse to the barn he gallops
toward what he wants—the kiln, the clay, the glazes,
his life as an artist.
Wisdom of eleven years ignores the cleared path,
creates its own way through drifts and patches of slush
to the studio
where the searing heat of the kiln is matched
by what burns in his young body,
the bright glazes fired in his eyes,
the clay formed in his hands.

May I live to see the arc
of this meteor, the blaze
of light as it strikes the atmosphere

Nikolski

Dec. 4, 1999 — Saturday.

I HAD THE USUAL PLEASANT HASSLE GETTING here. Two trips to the airport yesterday in Anchorage and both flights canceled due to weather out here. When I heard what the weather was like I was glad the pilot didn't attempt it. I am always afraid I will be with some cowboy pilot who thinks he has to try.

Better weather today, and it felt so good to be back in Dutch, even if it is only a stop on the way to Nikolski. The harbor as gorgeous as ever-fresh snow and that clear Aleutian light I love so much.

When we checked in at Anchorage they told me they were heavy and one of my three bags had to be labeled to be left behind in case they were over-grossed. What a decision— clothes? food? books? Reluctantly I chose books. I laughed when I got to Dutch. The two that arrived were clothes and books. The flight to Nikolski delayed so I checked my two bags and walked to Eagle Grocery to buy more food. It began to snow and blow but I made it back $45 poorer and waited. They assured me my food would be on the 4 p.m. jet from Anchorage, but we loaded about 3:45. By then it was really snowing and we sat at the end of the runway with snow collecting on the wings while my week's worth of food circled, hoping to get in. And we sat and sat. We finally taxied back in where they brushed the wings, after which we were off, minutes before my supplies landed. PenAir promises me they will deliver my supplies on Monday. Of course that's "weather permitting," and from watching the weather shows, I know a big storm is moving in.

We flew down to Nikolski at 500 feet over water, which makes me nervous on floats and we were on wheels. I loved it, though, because I could see all the beaches. We cut across about where we paralleled Chernofski on Unalaska to Umnak, now off the right wing. Finally saw the base of Mt. Vsevidof, and the runway with horses off to the left. Then I could see all the way to the Islands of the Four Mountains—beautiful!

Agrafina and her husband, Scott, 4-wheeled my stuff to the clinic and I walked. It felt so good to be here. Oh, yes, saw Val and Pauline Dushkin at the grocery in Dutch. They won't be back until I leave—too bad. Scott wanted to know if I had remembered my gun because he knows where the mallards hang out. He says he will lend me one and that his dog is a wonder. I would like to go, even if I can't hit anything with a non-fitting loaner gun.

Water is in short supply and it all has to be boiled. I haven't heard what the contaminant is. I have water stashed all over the house—kitchen and bathroom. Glad I showered before I left. I am dutifully boiling everything that touches my lips. I DON'T want to get sick!

. .

8:30 A.M. AND STILL DARK OUT, WITH THE one-hour time zone change. I am now on Aleutian/Hawaii time. And what it is, is time for breakfast.

The only other village lights on are in St. Nicholas church. The edges of the blue roof show through the snow, and the building is looking beautiful once more. The restoration scaffolding is at the far end. I must go look at the interior. Barbara Sweetland Smith, a friend from Anchorage who is attempting to get all the Russian Orthodox churches in the Aleutians restored, must have had a hand in this. I really want to talk to her about this project.

Good heavens! Now I see a man working over at the church. I will have to don my boots and see what gives. Who in the village is up at 9 a.m. and working? Perhaps a priest—

No, it is a crew of three from Anchorage. The head carpenter is an artisan from Surrey, England, and the work is financed by a congressional act restoring war-damaged buildings. Barbara probably did some creative writing for this one. The church is beautiful inside and I shall have to take pictures. I also want pictures of the horses grazing in the cemetery. Why didn't I take my camera?

12-5-99

SUNDAY—I WENT for a long walk along N. Beach Road and encountered blowing snow off and on. Finally found I could walk in the lee of the cliff for shelter. Not many birds, mostly harlequin. I came back about 5:30 p.m., and as I came across town Scott called out, "We're all having hot showers. Come on over."

Interesting, I thought, after our discussion of the water shortage and the fact that my bathtub was full of water for flushing the toilet if the village runs out of water. I came into the clinic to get a towel and unload my gear. I checked the phone messages. There were two from Agrafina saying they were having a big pot of *halibut chowder* and would I like to

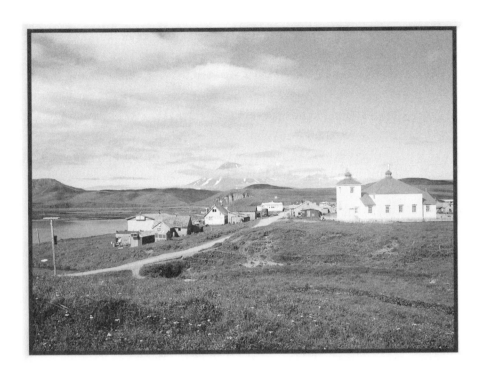

NIKOLSKI VILLAGE, *with* MT. VSEVIDOF *as dramatic backdrop.*
Photo courtesy of Daryl Moistner.

come for dinner. Hearing defects make life so interesting, even
if I had to leave the towel home.

The halibut was delicious. I drank a gallon of cranberry
juice as well, and caught up on news. Peat is back at the
Elbow Room and not doing any art work at all. (Sadness.)
Marlaine had a drowning death on her first charter for some
divers out beyond Adak. She ran afoul of the Navy bureaucracy in Adak—she had put the body in a skiff towed behind
the boat so as not to offend the living divers who probably
didn't want to share a bunk or smell him. No wonder I haven't
heard from her.

I got the name of a taxidermist, and Scott and I are to go
for a harlequin drake today. I just saw a flock of teal weave
up the creek behind the church, headed for the lake. A good
wind is pushing the sleet. I wish I had my double and my
dog, though Scott's Chessie, Whirlwind, is wonderful. Too
bad he isn't trained to handle so he could find birds he didn't
see going down. Scott is here—quick breakfast and we will
4-wheel to Pacific side for teal. Fat chance of my hitting one
of those fast, agile birds.

12-6-99

MONDAY—WHAT A day Scott and I had! We hooked the
trailer onto the 4-wheeler so that after hunting we could cut
driftwood on the beach and haul it back. I was grateful because that meant we would go slower and I would have a
more comfortable ride. The wind was really blowing by the
time we left. Sleet stung my face and I hid behind Scott's back.
The lake was almost frozen over so no birds there—on to the
beach we went. It was as he said—when the surf rolls in, it

stirs up the kelp on the edge, and there were hundreds of birds feeding. We crept into the blind and ended up with mallard, teal, gadwall, harlequin, and buffleheads—all good birds. Scott hunts in the usual Bush style of waiting until there are several lined up in a row so the shooter gets them all in one shot by sluicing. Shells are at a premium in the Bush so every shot must yield as many birds as possible. They are hunting for food, not sport. His poor dog never got the stimulus of seeing the bird fall. At first I thought he was dumb, with no drive, but that isn't it. He certainly isn't as "birdy" as my dog, Tig, but he is sure tough. We did get fliers on gadwall, and I was impressed to see him launch into that big surf and swim more than 100 yards. Just as he got there the bird dove under and Whirlwind dove right after it and got it!

I made a really long shot on another gadwall. Scott said he wondered why I was wasting a shot. Then the bird dropped. I was pleased, with a non-fitting gun. The shot was left to right, though, and I can usually hit those. I wouldn't have tried if it were right to left. We saw some gorgeous "pinners" but they didn't come close enough.

We packed up and trudged back to the 4-wheeler to go to the other end of the beach, where Scott had spotted a good log. He chain-sawed it into lengths and loaded it into the trailer while Whirlwind and I sat unproductively freezing in the blind. It began to warm and with the wind helping, most of the ice on the lake was gone. Big flocks of birds were resting in the middle. Sure would have been good to have Tig along. He would probably have fought (and lost) with Scott's dog.

. .

Dog Training

The first things a pup must learn are to sit and stay until released and then to come when called. The command may be either verbal or by whistle if the dog is away from its handler. The ability to sit, stay and come when called has real value in hunting situations. For instance, one might be duck hunting with others from a blind as a flock of ducks comes into the decoys. The hunter shoots one bird, which drops; if the dog leaps to retrieve it, as every ounce of DNA tells it to, it may not see the second or third bird shot. Perhaps one of these later birds is merely crippled, able to dive or swim to safety. The hunter will direct her dog to that bird first because it might otherwise escape. When the dog returns, the hunter will then line it up for the next bird she wants returned.

Before hunting season we train using bumpers rather than birds. These are rubber boat bumpers about a foot long and two to three inches in diameter, thrown to various locations. A short rope is attached to enable longer throws.

"Mark" means to observe and remember where each bird falls. Experienced dogs will plot a course over the terrain as they mark the fall.

Once the dog is steady to shot and flush, the next phase of training, called "handling," begins. The dog does not see the bird go down and thus has no genetic urge to retrieve it. This is called a "blind" rather than a mark and must be entirely taught because of that lack of genetic urging. The hunter places a bird without the dog observing her. Then she "sits" her dog, pointing toward that spot. Usually the cue "dead bird" is given, so the dog knows that there is a bird somewhere and that its handler will guide the way. On the command "back," the dog begins to run. If the dog is off course, the handler blows a "sit" command on the whistle. The dog stops, sits and looks toward the handler, watching for directions. If the handler wants the dog to turn to its left and go straight back, she will raise her right arm vertically and shout "back." For a 90-degree right turn (to the dog's left as it faces her) she will point her arm straight out to the right and shout "over." When the dog absorbs this, the angles become more refined, with quarter backs (45 degrees) and quarter "ins."

This isn't so hard on flat ground, but when dense, prickly shrubs, fallen trees, or rivers—or as in one memorable case, a fast-flowing riptide past an island—are added, handling to retrieve is a real challenge.

—N.E.S.

Home to thaw out. I made tea for myself (laced with a little vodka), put on dry clothes (lots of them) and tried to resurrect my harlequin for mounting. It was shot through the beak and blood leaked onto the white feathers so doubt it is worth saving for mounting, but it will sure taste good. Scott promises me a good one before I leave, and I will look for a suitable piece of basalt for it to sit on as a bookend.

Very windy all night, shaking the house so I had trouble sleeping. Calm this morning so far. The church is beautiful with its blue roof. I think the crew has cut the Tyvec from the windows. They certainly work hard. I will try to take a few pictures this morning. I hope the plane gets in with my food. Maybe later I will phone Bill and Mae Ermeloff and make a house call, and take cookies.

What a lazy lout I feel. I just pulled Bill's chart to review before I make the house call. That done, I resettled at the kitchen table to renew myself with Boccherini in my ears, eyes full of Vsevidof out the north window and the restored church out the south window gleaming in the winter sun against the rolling brown and white hills to the west. The surface of my mind runs over Martha Grimes with her wonderfully likable characters while the rest of my mind grapples with all else. It is so right to be here now. Feel like asking Peat to rent his house to me so I can live here with Tig and dig in the mess of my life. I'm still getting over the very difficult loss of Claire last August. Her death wasn't for lack of trying to survive, and she was filled to the brim with possibility. I won't ask Peat, of course, but it is nice to contemplate.

12-7-99

TUESDAY—I WAS IN a funk all last evening because the flight got in but my groceries did not. I really have enough food but did want the homemade cookies and the orange juice. I went to bed early and slept well. Now I just went to the store to stock up and Nick said the flight with my groceries should be in within the hour! A huge low is moving in so hope they beat it here. I bought a box of 12-gauge shells for Scott to partially repay for the great trip. I think he went out to slaughter a steer for winter meat yesterday. That should keep him busy. I hope he knows to keep it hanging for a while.

The man at the store told me again about the "nests" of trout they find in the winter. He told a charming story of looking for the "nest" with his mother and his aunt. They found an area of overhang which the fish hide under, and he jumped on it to check for the swishing sound of trout. The whole bank caved in when he jumped and there was a "blue stream of fish going out." They had no net so his aunt used her sweater for a net and got a lot of them. My mental picture is wonderful. I can feel their glee even now.

Off to see Bill and Mae. Nick will deliver my groceries if they come.

. .

HAH! I KNEW IT WAS TOO GOOD TO be true. The plane has come and gone—alas, no groceries. I like PenAir less and less.

The home visit went well. Then I went down to see Scott, who was hanging his beef in the smoke house. (He shot the fox that was getting in with his ducks, so his meat should be safe.) We will go before daylight for ducks. Wish I had my facemask. Hope I remember to take the radio. Wind forecast for 55 knots—it ought to be wild. I have one good piece of basalt for a base for my duck. I wish I had eggs and bacon for breakfast instead of oatmeal. I want something that lasts. I will take sandwiches and tea this time.

Diabetic schoolteacher was here just now for a bad foot. He has a collar-button abscess which is trying to heal. I opened the neck for him so it shouldn't take long. He invited me to dinner tomorrow night at seven. I look forward to it. He has been in the Kuskokwim Valley for years.

Clinic closed—will go for a quick walk along the beach.

12-11-99

SATURDAY NIGHT—THE woman I replaced did not show up on the flight that got in on Thursday. She probably thought the flight wouldn't make it so didn't bother to try, but I know she didn't want to come home until later so she may have planned it from the beginning and I am very disgusted with her. She had better be there Monday! If I didn't have so much to do at home with all the pre-Christmas chores I wouldn't care. Foul weather yesterday with high winds and sleet. No one came to the clinic, and I didn't even go for a walk. I got some corn-bread mix from the grocery and had split pea soup and corn-bread for dinner. Candy bar for dessert. I took Whirlwind to the Coast Guard landing for ducks. With the west wind it should have been good, but it wasn't. I wanted to get a pic-ture of Whirlwind, though. He was gorgeous with the surf shooting in the air off the rocks behind him and snow collecting on his coat. I had left my camera in my carry-on bag when I thought I was leaving—drat. It would have been an even better picture with a bird in his mouth.

I had Kerrs over for dinner tonight. Cooked butternut squash I had wisely packed in with my books, plus scalloped potatoes, a can of green beans and the frozen bass they had given me. We ate it all, and it sure tasted good. They brought lemon juice for the fish so we all had lemonade. Now I am down to bacon, eggs, the rest of the corn bread and a can of tomato soup.

Tomorrow I plan to take a swing around the lake with Whirlwind and then go over to Pacific side. I found a small thermos here so will take hot sugared tea and the rest of my M&M's. I plan cornbread with bacon and eggs both for breakfast and dinner tomorrow with tomato soup for late lunch. I hope the plane and my replacement get in Monday. I only have one book left that I haven't read. Sure enjoyed *Evensong*.

· ·

POSTSCRIPT: The more I saw of Whirlwind, the better I liked him. There had been a ranch on Umnak, and we often encountered cattle on our walks. I noted that Whirlwind always placed himself between me and the cattle. I didn't ask him to, he just did it. Comforting if the bulls started pawing and hooking with their horns.

Scott's story of a seal hunt impressed me even more. He and Daniel Snigaroff had planned to hop in a skiff and hunt for seal. When the motor refused to start, they reluctantly decided there was no way to hunt without it. Oars just don't cut it. Then, because they needed the meat, they thought of Whirlwind. If they could spot a seal within rifle range from shore, perhaps Whirlwind would retrieve it. I laughed at this point of the story, because I know a seal is about the same size as Whirlwind, and I have seen retrievers struggle to retrieve a big Canada goose.

"No, no," Scott said, and pulled photos from his pocket. The first was of Daniel sitting on driftwood near shore, with his rifle, Whirlwind alert behind him. Then Daniel takes aim at a dark head far out in the water as Whirlwind stands to get a better look. Now I could see blood where the seal had been. Whirlwind has leapt into the bay to retrieve it. And he does! Here he comes, the seal firmly in his mouth, as he drags it through the kelp and surf up onto the beach. What a dog! Scott says he would rather retrieve seal than ducks.

. .

12-13-99

MONDAY—A gorgeous day but foul in Dutch, so the Anchorage plane didn't get in—nor the one from Dutch to here. I had given my remaining eggs to Bill Ermeloff. The store closed by the time I knew I wouldn't get out. I had pancakes for dinner tonight—just found an ancient Pop-Tart in the back of the cupboard so am having it and de-caf tea before I go to bed. Dear Sue Linford called and made me laugh. I called my boys for a chat. If I am still here I will call again tomorrow.

Nick brought my baggage back from the strip and I have no idea where two boxes are—one with the frozen harley (harley out here is not a motorcycle but a harlequin duck). I bet it is inside and thawing. Maybe I can get another in the morning. I picked Scott's loaner gun up for the third time. The furnace man loaned me his 4-wheeler. I faxed the drug order in to the hospital tonight so maybe I'll hunt in the morning.

Superbowl Sunday in Nikolski

Jan. 30, 2000

The sea is silent this morning—
no surf or bluster of blowing snow,
as the day waits to blossom.
Outlines of hills, a few near houses,
nervy fox tracks on the drifts
toward the duck pens,
the bright blue of the church roof,
all unfold before me as a gift.
I will use it to hike over to Pacific side
and pretend to hunt ducks,
watch the gaudy harlequins, the Steller's eider,
see the emperors on the rocks.

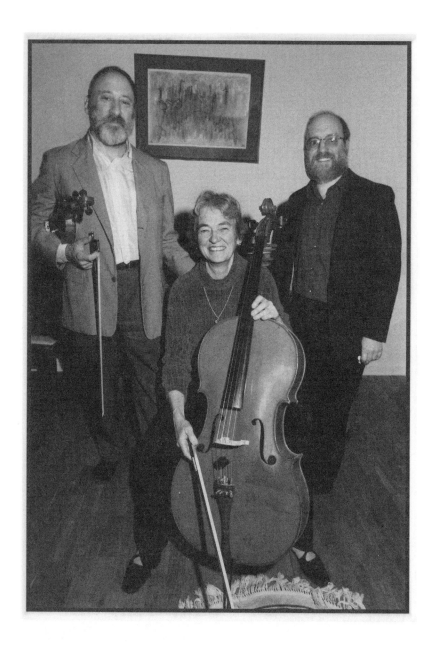

At home in Anchorage with PAUL ROSENTHAL *(left)*
and pianist DEAN EPPERSON.

Feb. 4, 2000 — Friday.

I AM TRYING TO GET HOME FOR THE Sitka Chamber music. At least I told Paul, my friend and the director, that if I wasn't there it was because I couldn't get back. After three days of dreadful storm it was beautiful in Nikolski yesterday. PenAir took care of everyone else first so by the time I got here to Dutch my jet had already left for Anchorage. I figured I would get out first thing in the morning but it began to storm again in the night. I had dinner with Marlaine and Axel at Cora and Milt's place. Cora and Milt are in Idaho for yet another hip replacement for Milt. They have torn down that dreadful cabana and built a decent home. It is decorated with all kinds of stuff from the ranch. Ann would have been delighted. It was an excellent visit. Marlaine took me to see her new sailboat on my way home (both entering the car from the driver's side). I like the boat, and we plotted a 10-day sail to the Islands of the Four Mountains next July. She will take Ann, me and two others. I would love to do it. I hope I don't shoot my wad on Botswana, where my friend Diddy has invited me for a horseback safari that I hope will keep my thoughts off Claire's death. I am beginning to think that one doesn't "get over" such things, but just gets used to them.

Up early and by 11 a.m. it was clear that all three flights were canceled. I called the APIA clinic to see if they wanted me. Did they ever! Irene came right over and bought me lunch and I worked hard all afternoon. One unfortunate woman had a large pleural effusion. The aides hadn't been able to convince anyone that she needed to be seen in Anchorage. We faxed the info out and she may bump me on the flight out.

After work Irene took me to Nicky's, where I bought chopsticks and two books, and then I had dinner at Tino's where the waitress recognized me and told me how good I was when she was pregnant 8½ years ago. Always makes me feel good.

I had made an appointment with the "Dutch Masseuse" (Juliette) for 7 p.m. and was so glad to see her. She is much the same as ever, and the massage was great, of course. That was my present for missing the Sitka music. She drove me home—in a truck with no wheel well. I am happily listening to Boccherini cello concertos on my swell headset with superb sound. I plan to sleep early and spend the day wait-listed for every flight. I'm confirmed on the 4:47 p.m. but that doesn't mean a whole lot. Just called my friend Karen to let her know what's happening.

Now the Boccherini is to the slow movement, which is wonderfully melodic and I think I could learn to play it. Even trying to play it would be a joy.

I must be mellowing—I'm not bothered by this delay at all. Having my son Ben and his wife, Janelle, in my house keeping it from freezing may have something to do with that. They came up from Oregon to take care of Claire's younger son, Cornelius, and haven't bought a house yet. Storm is going to college at UAA and living in the dorm plus hanging out at my place.

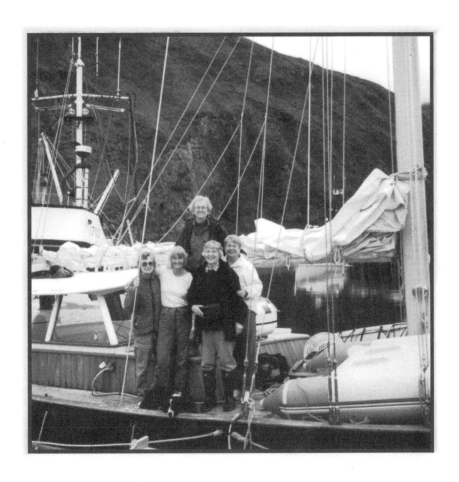

ABOARD THE *SPIRIT*, JULY 2000, *with (in front, from left) my sister,* ANN
BOYNTON; MARLAINE SKELLY, *the skipper; and friends* MARGARET SHARROW
and SUE LINFORD. *(Marlaine's one-man crew,* AXEL ALLAN, *was the photo-
grapher.) Ahead of us was a magnificent weeklong trip around Unalaska
Island—Kashega, Chernofski, Makushin; Cannery and Protection and
English bays; Udagak Strait. Margaret's son had said, "You can't go out
there—that's where the Mother of Storms is." Margaret's response
summed it up for all of us: "What an opportunity!"*

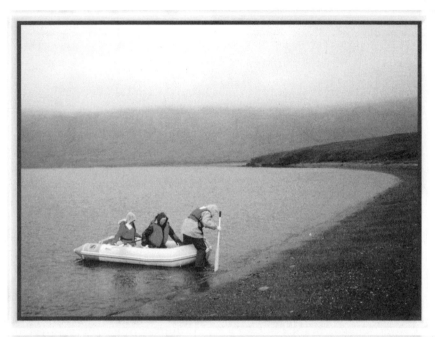

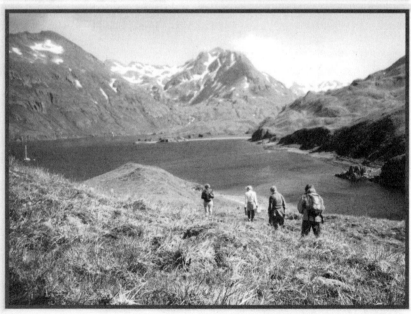

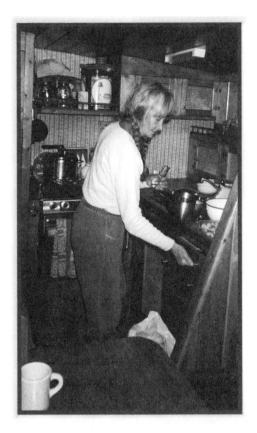
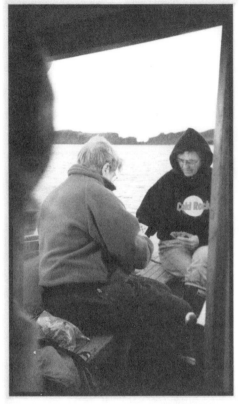

THE OUTBOARD WE HAD COUNTED ON *wasn't working till week's end,
so most trips to shore were by paddled Zodiac raft—a feat in any wind,
and this is, after all, the Aleutians. But even with challenges from buzz-
diving eagles ("Put your packs over your heads or you'll get scalped!")
or territorial bulls, as at Chernofski, the splendors ashore made up for
any rough water and weather. In the galley Marlaine produced 4-star
omelets and scones and salads and salmon croquettes (from the reds
we caught with a gillnet in a stream at Makushin). And at quiet times
Sue tried unsuccessfully to teach me to play euchre. This trip,
we agreed, could be a book of its own.*

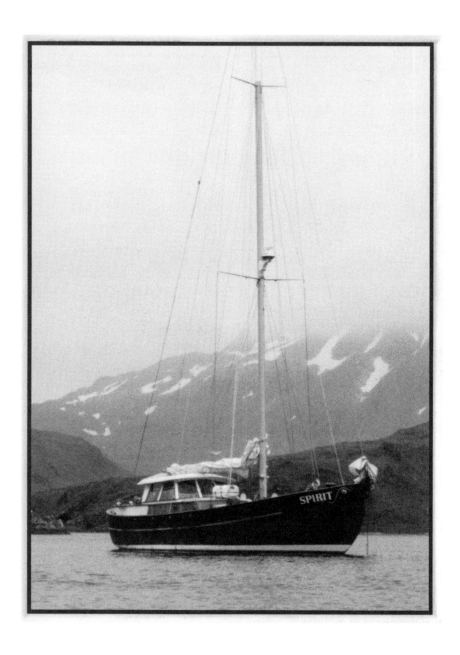

St. Paul

Oct. 14, 2000 — Saturday.

THIS TIME I'M IN THE UPPER UNIT IN the clinic building next to the King Eider Hotel, with a very different view than the apartment over the clinic at the other end of this building. The windows are high and I can see only the tops of the dunes, the houses on the crest above the cemetery, and the Bering Sea out beyond East Landing. As always, mist hovers over all.

I got in yesterday in the late afternoon. I had to get up at 4 this morning for a dislocated right shoulder on a very drunk man. I put it right but he was back at 8:45 having stretched and dislocated it again. I repeated the process and taped it to stay in place for a few days. I hope it works.

No wind so I may go for a walk after cello practice. Dear Reeve Aleutian Air let my cello ride in the cabin and I hand-carried it off, though when the wind caught it we nearly took off along the runway.

Now it is dinnertime, but I took care of a crush injury. A man was putting groceries into his truck when another man whose truck had no brakes slammed into him so that he was pinned between the two vehicles. Everyone says, "Oh, yeah, old _____ don't have no brakes on that rig—and he drinks, too." So casual.

Washington's Birthday

This day on the farm in Lynden
Cornie would be plowing the north forty,
cursing the wetness of the old creek bed
as he plods behind the horses while
I walk the furrow looking for arrowheads
left by some long gone tribe

camped along the creek
having set their nets for an early run of salmon.
The stumps he snags on the share
would be just leafing out,
dappling the clear running water
headed for Puget Sound.

My father would be digging his yearly
four foot deep trench for sweet peas
—horse manure, loam, horse manure, loam—
and the stems, when they came, would be long as bean poles,
holding blossoms big as hummingbirds,
their scent a start on heaven.

My mother would be opening a jar of peaches
canned in clear mason jars last summer
with their juices running down our arms.
The quick blanching and then the slip of the skins
to leave succulent flesh ready now
for bubbling cobbler with sugar and cinnamon
topped with fresh cream.

This day in the midst of the Bering Sea
I listen to the groan of this old building
as it leans against the wind,
a white stream of eternity past the window,
echoing, echoing.

St. Paul

Feb. 21, 2001 — Wednesday.

EASY TRIP OUT WITH PENAIR ON THE 18TH—strange not to
have Reeve, but the company retired. This was a small plane
so no chance to bring my cello. The flight left at 10:45 a.m.,
landed in Dillingham on the Nushagak River for gas, then St.
George Island in a snowstorm and finally, St Paul around
3 p.m. Ann and Suzanne, the two PA's here, are going out.
Suzanne fell on the ice and broke her leg bone (tibia) last
week. I wish I had brought my crampons instead of snowshoes. There is hardly any snow.

I came in on Sunday, so took a walk out to Reef Point to
reintroduce myself to the wildness, gusting winds, and pounding surf. Crabbers anchored in the lee of the reef, foxes sneak-
ing looks at me. I felt good after lugging all my books, tapes
and food up those stairs to my atelier.

Monday was Presidents Day, another day off. I worked on
poems, read, listened to music and wrote letters. Then I got
the Suburban and drove out to NE beach and walked. It was
a gorgeous day. The rookeries seem barren with the seals
gone, but it smells better. Caribou had herded up on either
side of the road on the way out.

Yesterday the PA's and I paid for the three-day weekend.
We worked hard all day, and Georgia was off sick so we were
short-handed. Then the x-ray machine quit on us. We had the

usual array of orthopedics with sprained ankles, lacerations, a possible fractured patella, head injury, and fights. We also had obstetrics, with a VBAC (vaginal birth after Caesarian section) due in a month. I enjoyed it but was tired at the end of the day. Karen sent a jigsaw puzzle out. My kitchen table is full of books, typewriter, tapes, and small boom box plus I write there, so I used the luggage table, which is about one inch larger than the puzzle. I color-coded the pieces and stuck them on cookie sheets and chairs. It worked well. I am sorry that I'm done with it. Maybe I'll take it out to the elders' home and exchange it for one of theirs. Or maybe they don't do such nonsense.

I saw Peter Schewe today and talked to him about being middleman for Paul Rosenthal from the Sitka Music Festival, who wants to give a brief concert here. Peter seemed to be delighted—said he would see about using the high school for the performance.

2-22-01

THURSDAY—I JUST got back from having dinner with Rick, the medic on the *Arctic Star*, a processor for Icicle. This isn't Casablanca and he isn't Humphrey Bogart—drat—but we had fun anyway. He even came to pick me up, in a ratty old truck that had to be left running while we ate lest it not start again. We viewed the ship's sick bay, and in the cafeteria the women were so glad to see me. I thought, "Oh, they're glad a woman doctor is around." Hah! They thought I was a replacement and they could go home. It was a good meal, and I didn't have to cook it myself.

Today was another busy day. At least the x-ray machine works now. I got cases back where I just used clinical judgment and the good physical diagnosis June Klinghoffer taught us in medical school. I was gratified to see that I got 100% right.

I checked an 18-year-old crab butcher whom I had seen yesterday with a stertorous heart murmur, which is drastically different today. I sent him out and hope he does OK. He had 100% O_2 stats with shortness of breath—does that make sense? I'll probably never know. It didn't sound like crab asthma.

This is the end of crab season and they are gearing up for cod, so things remain busy. I could shoot one kid who fell off his 4-wheeler. I told him no gym or basketball because he had torn a ligament. At 2 a.m. his parents called because he had played basketball and now the knee was swollen and sore. How come he didn't mind? Now he will have to go Outside for surgery.

I wear hearing aids and was asked to see a man who wouldn't tell the front desk why he was there. Those illnesses are always sexual. In the privacy of the exam room I asked why he had come. "I got VD," I heard him say, so I asked him about painful urination, or urethral drip or any rash. He looked at me sort of funny and said, "I got rectal incompetence." The plot thickens! I think VD, rectal "incompetence" —he must be gay and engaging in the wonderful pastime of "fisting." I asked about trauma, which he denied, so I asked if he had diarrhea, thinking that was why he couldn't control his stool. He kept saying he had "rectal deficiency." I'm wondering where he got all the correct medical terminology. Most guys just say, "My ass ain't workin'." Finally he says really loud, "I got E-D, Doc, E-rectile deficiency." Poor man—I gave him his precious Viagra (from which ads he probably got the terminology). Ten of the little rascals cost more than $100. I guess he forgave me because he came back a few days later to have his ears cleaned out.

The weather has become clear for a few days so I have walked my favorite close beaches. One day I took the Suburban (after filling it with 35 gallons of gas for $83!) way out to NE Point and walked out there. Sometimes ivory can be found on the beach. I'm usually so busy thinking that I never find anything. If it clears off this afternoon I'll see how far I can get on the west road. Still hardly any snow and me with those snowshoes.

Time for yoga—I made a schedule for myself. Wind is blowing rain on the windows so there is no temptation to skip it.

2-27-01

TUESDAY—I HAVE been up half the night coping with domestic violence. I couldn't sleep after I got home so am pretty bleary-eyed. Think I'll take a nap instead of eating lunch, which reminds me that Rick took us all to lunch at the *Arctic Star* yesterday. I had a real cheeseburger and skipped the pig's feet in some kind of sauce.

Mardi Gras tonight and I hope the village is unaware of it. I look forward to Lent, when for some reason there is less night call.

3-2-01

FRIDAY—THE EVENING is perfectly beautiful, with fresh snow, bright sun and no wind—and I am so pooped I didn't even go for a walk after work. I had a patient with bad crab asthma in overnight. He weighed 400 pounds, which didn't help a lot. I checked before I went to bed, and Pauline stayed with him, but I still slept poorly and then dear Alexay came in today about 10 a.m. in severe congestive heart failure. He had four plus edema everywhere—the works. I had a hunch he would respond and not need medivac, but it still is worrisome. Socked him with big doses of Lasix IV, nebulized him with the usual, started oxygen and managed to carry it off. I'm too old for the old brinksmanship. I sent him home on room air with oxygen saturation of greater than 95%, which I thought miraculous. I will see him at 10 a.m. tomorrow. I like him and his family.

In the midst of all that, the papers from the sale of Claire's house came through on fax so I had to deal with getting a notary, faxing back, mailing originals—and Carlann, the incoming PA from Adak, called to chat. I told her to call back on Monday. She no doubt thinks I'm rude.

The Air Force came today with their docs, medics and dentist. They made hay for a day and a half. Nice to have backup on the crab allergy, but the doctor is so cautious. He is a pleasant young man who gets out of the service in six months and plans to practice in Anchorage. He will do well even if he doesn't do obstetrics. It was wonderful to have the dentist, who worked 12- to 16-hour days. They left this morning on the Coast Guard C-130.

I have written three new poems—none worth much but some potentially OK.

3-3-01

SATURDAY—I AM AN old woman tonight! "Bach Violin Concerto in E" with Mutter is just right. (Oh, thank you, Harold Borofsky, for the wonders you have taped for me.) I have had a whole day of feeling incompetent for these huge tasks. Alexay is still in cardiac failure. His oxygen saturations are OK, but he hasn't lost any fluid pounds and still looks awful. We are out of IV Lasix. The weather bad so no flights. I have him on oral Lasix and started prednisone today. Meanwhile the gravida three, VBAC, is in early labor and due in 2½ weeks. The danger is that if allowed to labor, she may split her previous uterine scar and bleed to death in minutes. She looked at me with big eyes this afternoon and said, "I'm afraid to die." I can do as well as anyone out here to keep that from happening, but we have no blood.

This seems to match the obstetrical danger I faced one summer while working in Kenya. I was doing a caesarian section under ether anesthesia when the lights went out. They did not have a standby generator so casually lit kerosene lamps! Ether is extremely volatile and I was sure the patient and the rest of us would be blown sky high. It didn't happen and I was relieved but have never forgotten the episode. I hoped my VBAC would fare as well.

A disaster during the night here was that the husband of one of the village aides drank over the weekend and is in the clink for sexual assault—big fight. It makes me ill. I ache for his family.

I also cared for a serious nose-bleed (epistaxis), left nare. I saw the site but we have no silver nitrate that I can find to cauterize it. I packed it with gauze and added neosynephrine and sent him off. He was back in an hour with blood pouring from his right nare. Why? His blood pressure was normal. Too much aspirin? Who knows. I will never forget my first tough epistaxis—it is no laughing matter! I packed the right side as well and hope it stops. He is such a nice man. He doesn't want me to have to come out at night, and that worries me. In my mind I am threading string into his posterior nasopharynx to tie onto a big wad to block it off. Maybe I should have done that to begin with.

There is more but I don't feel like chronicling it here. Then my relief due in tomorrow is stuck in Adak in a snowstorm and may not get here on the 8th. I called my friend Karen to cry on her shoulder. She was wonderful as usual—appropriately concerned, didn't try to solve my problems (how could she?)—just there. She doesn't leave for Halibut Cove until Friday so if I get in Thursday she will pick me up. I look forward to that.

3-8-01

THURSDAY—SUPPOSEDLY, today I depart. High winds, of course. After Monday's debacle the week improved dramatically. Everyone arrived at work Tuesday with smiles. There had been fog in the night. Apparently that is like crocus, a harbinger of spring. "Winter is over!" they said. The epistaxis did well. I even dared unpack him. Alexay lost 10 pounds of fluid and was so happy—as was his family. The VBAC got out on the plane. The spelling bee at the school was well attended.

Good weather for my evening hike for two whole days and I got Karen's letter yesterday afternoon. (It took 11 days.) Then Carlann got off Adak yesterday. I rejoice. It is time to go home and rejoin the fray. Enough of this "forcing the hand of perception," as Eavan Boland would say.

3-9-01

FRIDAY—"THE BEST laid plans." When Carlann didn't come on Tuesday as planned, APIA forgot to change her reservations, so she was standby yesterday and couldn't get on. As a result, here I am. It is probably a good thing. Now I am standby for Sunday, Tuesday, Thursday, and confirmed for a week from Sunday! I might as well relax. They want me in Nikolski in April and May, but I have commitments at home so will probably turn them down. It is too soon after this trip, plus it is breakup time, when I worry about leaving my house unattended.

3-10-01

SATURDAY—I WENT to a basketball game last night ($2.00) to watch the St. Paul Islanders play the Raptors and then the Tribal Council vs. The Outcasts. They played pretty good ball and had one woman on each team. "Our" Samantha scored a bucket. Lots of my ortho patients were out there "playing through their pain." I liked knowing the players. They are all ages, gray hair through high school, and they take it very seriously. No night calls, thank goodness.

Atka

Feb. 27, 2002 — Wednesday.

I CANCELED MY CELLO LESSONS AND will miss the next concert to come out here. The plane took two tries to get in to Dutch, but we made it. Atka is not nearly as attractive as Nikolski— beautiful black sand beaches but they are dead. No birds or foxes, lots of eagles on the cliffs. I wish I had snowshoes or a kayak. The clinic is not well supplied. Dave Davelos, the wonderful PA-C from Dutch, is working on that, and I am making a list.

It feels good to be here, but I seem to be doing a lot of thinking and not getting anywhere. Maybe I will try collage-making with old magazines to find out what is going on with me. It worked in the spiritual discernment seminar I went to in Baltimore just before I came out here.

3-2-02

SATURDAY — A VERY windy day, and I am waiting for a boat with two injured men to arrive for airlift out. They were to have been here at 2 and it is now 4:30 p.m. It must be slow going in these big seas—even Nazan Bay is all chopped up. No walk this morning—I heard the wind howling so rolled over and went back to sleep.

I won $40 at Bingo last night after Spiridon blessed my new cards. I offered him part of the pot but he refused. I will

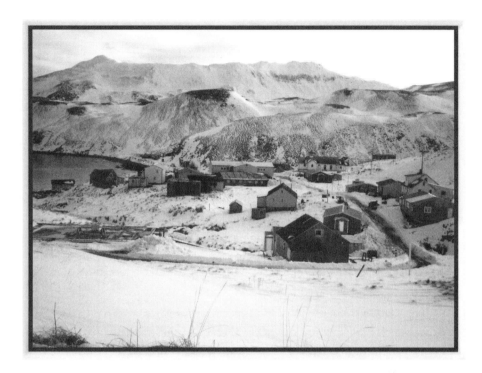

Atka village.

give mine to the church tomorrow. Spiridon is so interesting at age 72, with great stories of trapping out here in the islands. He was 11, cold and hungry and walking the beach with his uncle when a Coast Guard skiff came by and picked them up, took them aboard and warmed and fed them. His face glows at the memory. They offered to return him and his uncle home but his uncle said there were four others on the island and they had to stick together—so back to the cold beach they went. He said the store bought blue fox for $12 each and sold them in Seattle for $60–80, which sounds pretty normal for this screwed-up world.

I'm listening to Brahms and thinking of a book I brought along, The *Demon of Longing*, which incorporates Girard's premise that desire is what makes us human. The book is all short stories, weird but interesting.

3-17-02

SUNDAY—I HAD A wild trip back to Anchorage. We got out of Atka OK, thanks to a very gutsy pilot who landed way below minimums. Good GPS, I guess. We flew at 8,500 feet and in clouds the entire way. I was in the co-pilot's seat and thought we iced up pretty bad when we lost 20 knots of air speed, something I always keep my eye on. I felt better when I noted we had no loss of altitude. The boots (flexible rubber pads on the leading edge of the wings) worked to get rid of most of the ice on the leading edges. I was glad to get down in Dutch. The pilot made a nice one-wheel landing in a crosswind. Then we were stuck for three days in Dutch. At one point we all checked in and went through security and watched a jet appear through mist. He tried three times to land and couldn't keep on course. Bad wind shear, so he turned and left for Anchorage.

I had called the Oonalaska clinic to see if they wanted me to work, but Margaret Baldwin and a midwife were there so they didn't need me. I had lunch with Abi. She is retiring from Nicky's Place. Good to see her so happy. I couldn't reach Juliette. I ended up playing Kings in the Corner with Margaret and the midwife at the airport while we waited for the plane that finally made it in the next day. It was a hairy takeoff. One woman screamed at the usual 45–50-degree bank right after we cleared the end of the runway over the water. Fortunately we were high enough so the wing didn't hit the water. I thought the pilot was pretty good.

Letter from St. George

St. George 8-8-02 — Thursday

DEAR LINDA,

Fifteen minutes to the start of official office hours and I am at the dining table watching the wind in the thigh-high grasses on the east side. I would like to be able to see the water to the west, but my view toward the hills, at least a mile away, is decidedly better than at Atka, where dune grasses spread out and up about three feet from the only window.

So far, so good. It was the usual hassle getting out here, with a late start. I realized I had left my beloved jackknife in my pocket and was ready to turn back and check it as luggage when I found there was no security check—are terrorists interested in St. George?—so all was well. It does make a difference when you don't have to take your shoes off or be "wanded." We went nonstop to St. Paul and then had to wait to see if it would clear enough to get in to St. George. I sat in the sun on the steps of the terminal with other passengers and read Adrienne Rich with a background of murmured Aleut which I love so much. We finally left, and coming in I could see the island nestled into the sea with an ermine ruff of clouds over most of it—only the center with the airstrip was clear. Sheer cliffs on what shoreline I could

see. None of the long clear beaches I wander on St. Paul. I
was met by Georgia, and joy of joys, all my baggage came,
and her teenage son who had just learned to drive was our
chauffeur on the five-mile trip to the village. We had gotten in
just before six, which is when the store closes, but I managed
to get coffee and cereal for today. Instead of per diem, I get
to run a chit at the store. It seemed at least as well stocked as
at St. Paul. The clinic and quarters are a short walk away.
Nice spacious quarters—two baths, one with tub, one shower,
cable TV and video set-up. There is a huge freezer plus a
regular refrigerator and a non-working dishwasher. Majestic
by village standards. Interesting décor—lace curtains, mauve
sconces. I am comforted by the thought that dyslexia in
plumbers is the norm for the islands—as in the Aleutians, hot
and cold water are universally reversed.

There are about 190 souls here. (Did you know that
when filing a flight plan, you're asked not how many
passengers are on board, but how many souls?) Coming over
the last hill into the village there is a stunning view of the sea
splashing on the shore, waves filled with seals. The air is
swarming with white birds against the oh, so blueness of the
water. The village perches upon the upthrust of land, the
white church rampant. After settling in I walked back out
and took a few pictures. One never knows when the next sun
sighting will be.

More later. I have until tomorrow to get this into the
mail for the Sunday flight.

. .

Now it is Friday morning and I seem to be in a Beethoven mood—the late quartets to sleep on and the "Archduke Trio" now. I never know if my choices derive from inner or outer circumstances. I like St. George better and better, though, and that seems to fit with the music, which is beautiful and harmonious.

It is 6:30 a.m. and so much farther west that it is still almost pitch black outside. Of course that means it is light later here—nice because I was able to go for a long walk after dinner. I went east along the cliffs. I am cross at myself for neglecting to bring my bird book—so many and so beautiful. I love the smell of the sea, the sounds, the sight. I felt like your granddaughter Sophie—soaking it all in like a big sponge. It makes me feel larger, less empty.

The path toward the cliffs is not easy. Boulders are hidden beneath the growth. Lupine is in seed (I'll bring some pods home) and another blue flower is in abundance.

From the cliffs I could look down to the clear water to watch the seals and sea lions. They assume such luxurious and ridiculous poses, often with one flipper up like a sail. They are so liquid that I never quite know which part I am seeing. Thought of ballet and how arduous that road to perfection is in comparison with the effortless grace of these creatures. Claire studied ballet for years. I think she thought the discipline would somehow hold her together. Perhaps it did.

It was after 9:30 when I got home, and my darned Achilles tendon gave me fits. Once again I forgot to bring my brace (the cost of denial—Karen says it's my vanity). I iced

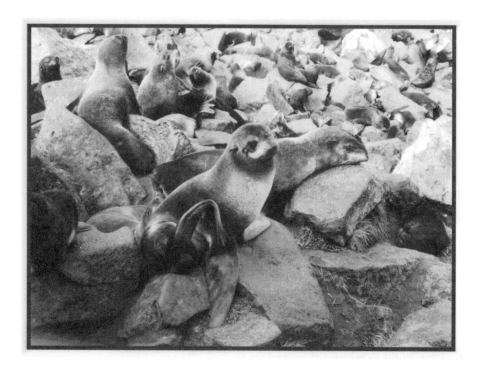

"SEAL HEAVEN," *as recounted in the story of* IGIADAX
discovering the PRIBILOFS.

my foot and made my own brace out of a thick toner box. Just the right width and I lined it with my good Patagonia long johns. I found some orthopedic straps to hold my foot in, and it worked fairly well. I can walk OK this morning.

I will earn my salary. The clinic is a mess, and I have to organize it. Stuff is piled everywhere. (Having seen my garage, you can imagine how bad it is for me to even notice it.) I was swamped and couldn't find anything I looked for. There has been only one PA here since June, and all the blood draws have piled up. I will attempt to corral people and get them done next week—on the mornings the plane comes in to take the samples out. The paperwork is the worst part, as in any government job. "Julie who knows everything" was kind enough to spend an hour with me yesterday to point the way. She is very intelligent and worked here for years until she got sick. I like her and will be pleased if I can remember all she told me—three copies of everything. I haven't even been to the post office to see what awaits me. Two huge boxes here that I thought were incoming drugs turned out to be expired drugs to be mailed out. What waste there is in isolated communities! At least someone had sorted them out. Perhaps they will be sent to Africa and sold for a fortune on the black market.

St. George feels entirely different from St. Paul—smaller, less hurried. I don't get the undertone of violence I get in Dutch or St. Paul. The patients are very funny and friendly. I love Aleut humor. I'm on to them, and it pleases them if I laugh when they make fun of me. So subtle that you have to be aware and expect it.

They have told me of the good beaches on "the other side" —where they always seem to be. I think the island is only a few miles wide so I will pack a lunch and hike over there this weekend—packing a radio, of course. I have let it be known that I want to go halibut fishing so will see what transpires.

I had best eat breakfast and get on with my onerous task. Oh, meant to tell you that the Beer Hall hours here are Monday–Friday 5 p.m. to 5:30 p.m. (not a misprint), closed Saturday and Sunday. Isn't that great? There is gym 7–9 every night and Bingo on Saturday. Who has time for reading? (Now my music is Mendelssohn's "Italian" with Pablo Casals.)

8-10-02—Saturday. TODAY IS A PSALM 139 DAY—"If I take the wings of the morning and dwell in the uttermost parts of the sea—." I once visited Lindberg's grave in Hawaii, and that was on his headstone. Anyhow, I am about to take the wings of this morning and hike to the other side to roam the beaches at the uttermost part of the sea. Naturally it is raining and I wish I had brought a thermos for hot tea. I could stay home and read and see how the weather is tomorrow or perhaps call Georgia to see if I could borrow a thermos. No, I don't dare call her at this hour. No one gets up before noon on weekends. You can see that I am procrastinating.

It was so hot in here yesterday that I propped the clinic doors open as well as all the windows. Mark Merculief really laughed when he came in—said the foxes would move in before I could blink. They quickly pee on everything to mark it as their own, and I can tell you there isn't much that is more unpleasantly pungent than fox urine. My mental picture of returning from lunch in the quarters to foxes in the clinic was not one of delight. Hot or not, the doors stay closed.

Enough. My morning dose of Boccherini is completed. I will mix up some tuna for sandwiches and go. If I find a glass ball it will be yours.

8-11-02—Sunday—Mother's birthday. AND NO GLASS BALL. What a trip! Toughest I have ever been on out here. Today will definitely be a reading day because I can hardly move. I have made it to the coffeepot and my music (Ofra Harnoy with the Vivaldi cello concertos) but that is all. From here I can see the path I climbed up the hills. It makes me shudder. The path disappears into boulders on the top and I felt like Moses wandering in the wilderness. Finally got up high enough to see where I didn't want to go (over a steep cliff), so tried to head for the beach where there was no cliff. Hand over hand most of the time. Then I fell badly on my back which knocked the wind out of me. I think the apple in my backpack saved me from a broken rib—applesauce—and the protruding stone missed my camera as well as the ever present radio.

I got within about a half mile of the beach and knew if I ever got there I would never be able to climb back up. I took a picture and ate my lunch. Then a thick fog descended and all landmarks disappeared. Fortunately I had the compass that never has left my backpack since I got caught on Chickaloon Flats with an incoming tide while duck hunting. I tried to take a less difficult route home. I felt secure with the compass, and after a couple of hours glimpsed the Russian cross I had seen on the way in, appearing in a ghostly fashion through the mist. I got home about 6 p.m.—too tired and not in the mood for either church or Bingo. I took a shower, ate an enormous dinner, iced my foot and went to bed.

The ceiling is much higher today and the plane ought to get in—if it stays high, that is. Onward with breakfast and then Adrienne Rich. What was I doing in the '70s? Ah—that was when I got divorced.

Now it is afternoon and Georgia stopped by to pick up her son's meds. I asked about the "beach trip." She said, "Oh no, you can't get down that way." Something I had figured out. She said you go up on the high cliff and there is a goat trail down and the whole trip takes only an hour and a half! Oh, well, maybe next Saturday. I am not about to attempt it today.

· ·

LATER: I COULDN'T STAND MY MOOD or my self any longer so glued things together and hiked out the road to the rookery. It was very pleasant and Bone, the EMT, drove by and stopped to chat. Said I could go past the signs to the seals. He also said no one had been to the searched-for beach this year and the path was overgrown. What path? Nice friendly man and maybe I will get him to move the huge boxes of meds at the post office. (Bone is short for "T-Bone," the name he was given because he's always looking for bones and other artifacts.)

· ·

Monday evening. WHAT A GLORIOUS DAY! Clear sun all day with only a few scattered high clouds. Not even any wind, more like a breeze. And I made progress at the clinic. I also decided to do all the blood draws on Wednesday morning. Thought I would organize it into three tiers of one hour apiece so no one would have to wait very long. I had the sense to ask Julie what she thought. She is so tactful: "Well, you could do it that way." She would have them all just choose when to come between 8 a.m. and noon and let chance take care of it They all get to visit that way, she says, and no one seems to mind waiting. I have so much to learn—or is it unlearn?

Bone may take me halibut fishing next weekend. They are very scarce this year, however, so don't start drooling. He told me some of the cliffs here are over 1,000 feet high. Pretty skookum!

I picked mossberries on my walk tonight after finding a wondrous patch. They aren't blueberries, but when in Rome. I will try them in pancakes tomorrow.

It pleases me that on my walks all the little kids want to know who I am and then gravely tell me their names— Serge, Nikolai, etc., and then tell me how they feel sick or sore. It is the seriousness that tickles me. I saw five fox kits out playing tonight—pretty well grown but still cute, very quick but quite tame and let me get about 10 feet away. They are living in a culvert just at the edge of town.

. .

Tuesday night. "JUST BEFORE THE BATTLE, MOTHER"—I am set up for the on-slaught of blood drawing. I do fine as a phlebotomist, it's the paperwork and finding boxes, tubes and equipment that swamp me. Then I have to get them all agitated, spun, cooled and on the airplane—if it gets in. Today I tracked down all the patients who needed blood drawn. We will see how many show.

Bone brought me a map of the island and showed me a closer beach, so I trudged off after supper. I saw some wonderful birds, and the seals put on a show. I was surrounded by foxes on the way home. I think I was too tired to enjoy it much. Got back here about 10 p.m. and will soon be in bed.

8-14-02—Wednesday. EARLY MORNING and pitch-black outside. I plan to do all the blood draws today—three months worth—and I am braced for it. I couldn't sleep last night thinking of all the congestion in the workspace. Empty boxes all over, no place to move, and I can't get to storage spaces.

. .

*L*ATER: HAH! THE VILLAGE MADE SURE to send the most difficult patient in first to see if I was any good. They are so smart. She had burn scars on both arms from her shoulders all the way down to her fingers. What a test! I slid a 23 butterfly (very small bored needle with two little paper handles to hold it by) into the one opening I could see and got two full tubes! I was off and running. The "grump" from the store said, "You're good, the best," and spread the word so that even some that weren't on the list came in. I ran out of forms, of course, but didn't care. It was fun—I couldn't miss. It took until almost three to get them wrapped and boxed with all the right forms (I hope). Four boxes full, barely on time for the plane, which did get in. Before I leave on Sunday I will try to catch the slippery ones who avoided it today.

I drew blood on the nice man named Bone. I had seen him out walking two nights ago. He "keeps track" of the reindeer and also searches for lost cheechakos like me. He said there is no radio communication from "the other side," which I had suspected. Now I am really glad I got back from the Garden Cove trip without incident. I think of him and his minute knowledge of this island—Elizabeth Bishop and her geography. It's all the same? That has to simmer.

I am domestic tonight and made cornbread, plus did the wash. I went early to bed, without my usual walk. I am so glad things went well today and can hardly wait for time to get into my clean bed.

8-18-02—Saturday. WHAT A GREAT DAY! After getting up to fix a busted nose and laceration at 4 a.m., I slept until 10 and had great pancakes with the mossberries I had picked, plus sausage. I saw a patient with an immunization reaction and checked the post office for mail. Then I cleaned the desk and set off for Garden Cove—found the right path and got on the beach. I found an aerie for myself where I sat between two beaches and watched foxes and seals and surf scoters on the beach. I also saw and heard a winter wren chirping away. Restorative. Then, as I listened to a Schumann tape of "Quartette in E flat" and then the Quintet, also in E flat, I looked up the opposite cliff and saw a whole herd of reindeer outlined against the sky! What could be finer than birds, seals, foxes, surf and reindeer? The round trip took six hours with leisurely walk and "sitting time."

After I got home T-Bone brought some halibut by. I would really like to get to know him and his wife better. We seem to speak the same language. Now, to bed. I will pack up in the morning and see if any blood draws show.

8-19-02 — Sunday. THE ENTIRE VILLAGE is gone in the mist and I am absolutely alone here with only near grasses visible. I wonder what the strip is like. It could be clear. I will wait until about one and call PenAir to see if they're coming. I find I'm ready to go home and at the same time won't be too upset if the plane doesn't get in.

Love,
Nancy

Canceled Flight

I'm supposed to be on my way to St. George.
Instead, I'm in a secret country
known only to myself,
cut off from everyone.
Even my dog is gone to friends.
The beauty that surrounds me
belongs only to me.
I am sated with the gold of the birch leaves,
the sheen of a glossy lake,
nuthatches and chickadees at my feeder,
an ermine crest of snow on the Chugach Range.

Letter from St. Paul

Dec. 11, 2002—Wednesday.

Dear Linda,

It took four long hours to get out here, in a plane with no bathroom and military-style, non-reclining seats. It had no carry-on space at all, and a 12-inch aisle. The flight attendant was a wire basket containing water and Fig Newtons, stuffed under every third seat. We were at least spared the screening and searches of the larger world.

Once we got out of Anchorage it was a beautiful sunny day, with the tops of the Alaska Range sticking up above the clouds. I was on the sunny side and had on Sorels with felt linings, so my head and chest baked in the sun and my feet, which would otherwise have been freezing, were toasty.

It was gorgeous here when we finally arrived. Phyllis and Simeon Swetzof met me. No wind, and sunny—they were agog. Said it had been so for three whole days. I hope it continues over the weekend so I can hike in comfort. I am in the sea-side end of the building this time, and it is the one I love. Ah, water!

Time for work—more later.

. .

The first patient was a 10-year-old with lobar pneumonia! Complete consolidation of the left lower lobe. I haven't seen one in years. She has been faithfully followed (but not had her chest listened to) for the last two weeks. She will go to Anchorage this afternoon. I hope we can get an IV started, but she is so dehydrated the veins are hard to find.

Later: Medivac on the ground—thank God for good weather. Her dehydrated level of iron in the blood (Hbg) was 10, so this is bad sepsis. So far she is not in shock. She is on her third bag of fluids and I have started her on Rocephin, so I think she will make it. Her Hbg is now down to 7 but that is from the hydration, not blood loss. Temperature is still 103.

Later still: And now she is on her way to Anchorage. We managed to get her on their stretcher without putting her into shock, so that is good.

12-16-02—Monday. Here I am at 5:30 a.m., all packed and looking at weather. Only snow showers here so the plane should get in. I checked on the 10-year-old with pneumonia. I was only able to get her lab work. She is still very sick, but alive. I think she will make it. It looks as if they transfused her with blood. I would have if I had had any.

Love,
Nancy

"He Hadn't Taken Anything"

I got called to ER tonight. The ambulance was bringing a 36-year-old male who on returning home after work had a sudden onset of pain and heaviness beneath his breast bone (substernal). When I walked in he was on oxygen by mask, lying on his back and completely unresponsive. His oxygen sats were 99, pulse regular at 130, BP 144/82, respiration 16, temperature 98 and blood glucose 257 (high).

I could hardly see him breathe, and he was extremely pale, but not sweating. The skin on his face was cold. His eyes were rolled upward and his pupils were dilated and not reactive to light. His deep tendon reflexes were 3-4 plus but equal bilaterally. Heart sounds were normal other than tachycardia. Lungs were clear bilaterally though he had poor inspiritory effort and minimal diaphragmatic movement. His abdomen was soft with no palpable organs or masses and normal peristalsis. I took an electro-cardiogram (EKG) which showed right bundle branch block. His chest x-ray was normal other than the high diaphragm because he couldn't "take a deep breath and hold it." I just timed the exposure for his shallow inhalation. His girlfriend assured us he hadn't "taken anything" and that his last alcohol ingestion was six beers the previous day. He had no vomiting or diarrhea.

The beloved telemed was down, the fax machine wasn't working, and we were in whiteout with gale-force winds, so medivac was not possible. The CBC machine was kaput, and I couldn't even get a hemoglobin. I got a line in and started a slow drip of normal saline. By this time we'd had him for about an hour.

We brought him back from the x-ray, and I noticed that he "helped" us get him on the exam table. I began to be able to see inspiritory effort, and he opened his eyes! His pupils were still dilated but he looked around and was no longer pale. I gave him 0.4 mg of Narcan IV anyway, just in case. Over the next half hour he became much more alert. I stopped the oxygen and his sats stayed high. His pulse remained around 100 with his respiration 18 to 20. I gave another 0.4 mg of Narcan after about 30 minutes. As he improved, he became very lucid and described the onset clearly.

He was home and suddenly had crushing substernal pain and almost simultaneously had loss of sensation in his left arm and leg, plus his chest felt like it had collapsed. He noted that he could move his legs and arms but could not feel them. There was slight nausea, but no vomiting. Next he could hear but was unable to respond. Now he sat up, walked around and in general became his old self.

This is more than previously undiagnosed diabetes. In spite of the denial of "taking anything," I bottled urine for drug testing and will send him to town on the next available flight. The response to Narcan is pretty indicative of some sort of drug overdose. I hope I never have to see another one. His coronaries may be able to stand it, but I am not sure mine can.

St. Paul

Aug. 24, 2003 — Sunday.

I WENT TO A PARTY WITH A GROUP of biologists on Friday. They were really fun to talk to. One is the "rat man" who tries to keep rats from jumping ship onto the island, where they will rapidly decimate the bird population. Another is an expert on oceans. It was fascinating to hear the real scoop on what oil does in oceans. It is much, much more lethal than we are allowed to know, but I do know that from what happened in Prince William Sound after the *Exxon Valdez* spill.

I also got to meet Larry Merculief, the appointed spiritual leader of the Aleuts. He was chosen as a young boy and brought up by the elder men. If I don't get out on the plane today, I will go to hear him speak at 2 p.m.

One of the women I met sea-kayaks. She told me of kayaking on the shallow beach where the mother seals teach their babies how to swim. (Shallow so the orcas can't get in and eat the babies.) When she and her friends kayak over there, the babies come up and very gently try to nurse on their fingers. She invited me out yesterday to kayak with the seals over in Lukanin Bay toward the airport. What bliss! They are such funny, lovely, graceful creatures. I was frightened at first when they rose, snorting right next to my paddle, but they don't try to turn the kayak over. They are just curious about what I am and what I'm doing. I had a wonderful time—and learned how to launch a kayak into the surf. Count on getting soaked!

Letters from Atka
(Dutch on the way)

Nov. 2, 2003 — Sunday.

Dear Linda,

I arrived in Dutch in grand warm weather, without wind, to find the airport full of surly people who had been waiting for days to get out—and only about a third of them made it. Ah, Dutch weather. A Native woman from Atka and I basked in the sun waiting for hotel pickup. Our plane won't be repaired before Tuesday, if then. So here we are, and I see my per diem going down the drain at a very rapid rate. $110 for the room here at the Grand Aleutian, and food is sky high. I have investigated Carl's over in Unalaska, but the rooms stink of stale smoke and the thin walls let all the bar noise in, plus the beds aren't much. They also cost $112 per day. Nuts! I have a nice mini home here on the second floor and use the coffeepot to make soup or heat canned stuff and the ice bucket to cool my yogurt or cheese. I have coffee and breakfast bars in the morning. What a cheapskate I am.

Halloween is wild out here. My favorite yard decoration is an inflated spider 6 or 8 feet tall whose legs flop and wiggle in the wind. A gorilla crouches on the roof above a witch next to a vat. Wonderful! One costume was a man with blood dripping from his neck and a small stuffed tiger attached. Tonight I had dinner (not out of the coffeepot) with a skinny guy who dressed as Arnold Schwarzenegger. He got really crude and squirted that string putty from his crotch whenever he saw a pretty woman. Holidays out here are much more fun than any in Anchorage. This man is a poet and said, "I've read your work in *Ice-Floe*." I nearly fainted with surprise.

I saw Abi again. She makes me laugh. This time she told me about the man who when he left town left a bag of dog food in his car. When he came back two months later the car was chock full of rats.

We went out to Morris Cove, and the wild horses were all there. The stallion was nasty—I didn't try to get too friendly. It was windy and raining so we didn't stay long. Abi has foxes near her house and they play with her cat. I would love to see that.

Today Juliette, the "Dutch Masseuse," called, and I was glad to put my EFM (Education for Ministry) lesson away and go for a walk. We drove up the valley to her new home, which is an old school building that has been moved to a patch of mud and gravel above the creek. I am glad I don't have to take on such projects any longer. I felt tired just looking at all that needed doing. It is quiet, however, and the scenery beautiful. We walked the bank up to the waterfall and beyond, discussing the state of humanity and testing what blueberries remained. The high blueberries were great but the low ones, yucko. Why? There were many fish in the creek and a lovely, deep pool under a rock with 15 or so 18- to 20-inch trout. Such clear water—such grace.

Juliette disclosed yet another secret—"Over that ridge is a shallow lake with black sand and water that is very warm in summer. A great place for skinny-dipping." Even I could climb that ridge for such joy. I'm glad to have sensuous friends. Which reminds me—the cryptoquote from the paper turned out to read "Platonic love is like being invited down to the cellar for a drink of ginger-ale." I laughed—my view, and always trouble.

PenAir called yesterday promising a plane today, so I am up early and have repacked the cooler and my bag ready to leap when they call. I will work at the clinic until then. I had a young girl with a terrible migraine last night. It was the only night call so far. On to Atka.

11-5-03—Wednesday night. WE MADE IT TO ATKA—in a Metro, no less. It is faster than the Navajo so took less than two hours and was an easy flight. The crew has "finished" the work they were doing in the quarters the last time I was here, and installed a washer and dryer. I think the dryer vents into the kitchen, which is interesting. I was dismayed to hear I was to share quarters with a woman engineer of some sort—a peculiar woman. I had forgotten that there are two bedrooms here. The second bedroom was full of building supplies the last visit. Anyhow, she keeps very much to herself, not sharing meals or space. When one of us enters the kitchen/living room, the other leaves. Fascinating. Suits me—I came to be alone, too.

The 4×2-foot piece of wallboard I worked puzzles on last time is still here, to my joy. I bought a 1,000-piece loon puzzle in Dutch. I have it set up on two filing boxes on top of chairs, just the right height. I am always at peace when I work puzzles. It is a welcome relief from the EFM demands of Hegel, Engels, Marx and Kierkegaard. I think philosophers take themselves much too seriously.

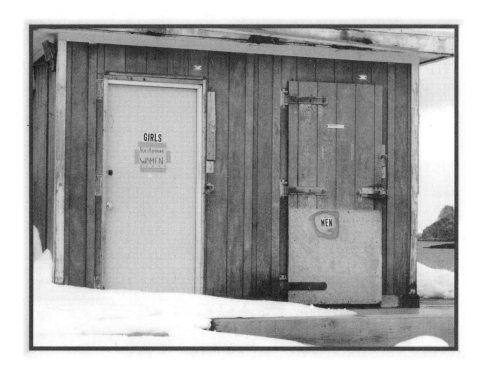

SOMEONE EDITED *these signs at* ATKA, *to the delight of at least half the population.*

Another sunny day today so after work I went for a walk along the cliffs to the south of town. Found a waterfall but couldn't get down to it before dark. I will pack a lunch and try this weekend. Oh, for a kayak here! Nazan Bay is a huge sheltered bay with lots of nooks and crannies.

Now it is Friday night and my phantom roomy has departed. (How did they ever make it in with 50-knot winds and clouds down to the deck?) I have found the tinny tape player and am happily listening to Bach violin concertos. I suppose I should be over playing Bingo but I'm not in the mood. I made a tasty butternut/apple bisque with coconut milk and Thai seasoning. How good it was! Tomorrow I will get wild and make butterscotch pudding with dates. I explored the store for ice cream and there is none, which is probably good because I've lost five pounds on this trip.

11-5-03 — Saturday. THERE WERE TO BE TWO flights out of Atka yesterday—the first, at 10:30 a.m., was a charter for the hydro crew (new water supply up that gorgeous creek I followed, with waterfall after waterfall), and for some reason I was assigned on that flight with them. It was also to take the luggage for the second flight as well as our flight. Tiel, the biomedical communications specialist (computer geek and my second roomy), was assigned to the second flight. He is new to the Aleutians so I warned him to keep his toothbrush. Naturally the flight was late, and we stood shivering out at the strip as the weather got worse and worse—the usual wind and rain. There is no "waiting room." We just try to stand in the lee of a shed. The plane finally arrived about noon. They quickly unloaded the passengers, then all the freight from cabin, wing space, and nose space, after which the ground crew put seats in for departing passengers and loaded the outbound luggage.

Finally, when I was almost a solid block of ice, we boarded. It was the Navajo this time. I sat directly behind the pilot so I could check his flying and the instruments. Off we went. I found to my horror that my seat was directly over the air vent, so that the outside air flowed around my feet and up under the seat. This was not one of those little nozzle things, but a 4×8-inch duct! I finally got a sweatshirt out of my carry-on and plugged about half the air flow, but it was still like sitting on an iceberg. By the time we got to Dutch the weather was about 100 feet off the deck, but that old boy wove his way through it and down, and we made it. I congratulated him and he said now he had to make a quick decision about whether to make the second run because it would be almost dark when he returned, and the weather would have gotten worse by then. When I picked up my bags I saw them gassing the plane, but I'm not sure it left. Poor Tiel. I warned him to learn to distinguish between inconvenience and catastrophe.

So I am here in Dutch, but still thinking of the wonderful walks on Atka, including that huge loop along the cliffs to the south and then up the "waterfalled" creek. I thought I would find the source, but every lake turned out to be just another contributor. I think the thing has hundreds of little feeder creeks. I tried to get high enough to see over into the Bering Sea near Korovin Bay but couldn't do it, so I looped back to the village from the west. Saw plenty of ptarmigan—Vita would have loved it.

The 11th [of November] was a holiday, so I rented a 4-wheeler and rode over to Korovin Bay. I wanted to beach-comb, but the tide was so high that I couldn't cross the creek and had to ride along the beach the other way. I kept stopping to explore, and on that black sand beach I found what looked like Easter eggs. They were multicolored rocks, unusual and so beautiful. I collected some for Sandy, Bruce's wife. I now refer to that area as "Easter Egg Beach." It was a wonderful day—started in sunshine but changed to snow and hail by the time I got out there. That didn't last long, though, and I had plenty of gear.

I had a good time at the clinic. Teresa is her usual helpful self. We made home visits with elders, which I love. I fixed Spiridon's feet again and heard a lot of village woes. There are only about 80 people at Atka now.

I really missed a good bet on halibut. I thought the season was over, but the hydro crew let it be known that they had run out of food. In response, the last boat in gave them all its small halibut plus the cheeks, usually thrown away. The hydro crew had been feasting for days—dang! I could have taken some home in my now empty cooler. Oh, well.

I was just called and have to be at the airport in half an hour. I will wait to tell of last night's dinner with Abi—the photos of the Arkansas bathroom, 40×12 feet with a pool and waterfall (of course, the "pool" is a converted watering trough and so far Mike has no running water).

Love,
Nancy

Perfect Vita

The series of Alaskan Dogs I Have Known starts with Pete, who was my husband's dog when we married. Then came Max, who so impressed the astronauts-in-training in Juneau, followed by Amy, loving but worthless as a hunting dog. I was so embarrassed by Amy that I never went hunting when anyone else could see how rotten she was. I have to add, though, that when we got stuck in the mud on Chickaloon Flats and had to spend the night, she was wonderful—unfailingly cheerful and a warm companion on a cold night. After Amy came Tigger, the first real field trial dog I had, and he was excellent at hunting as well. I have two Master National plates from running him.

When Tigger died I thought I would never have another dog. Club members kept asking if I didn't want to see so-and so's pups, but I always said no, I was done. Then someone showed me the pedigree for a breeding that really impressed me—plus I had found that hunting without a dog was no fun at all. When I was told I could have the pick of the litter I said I'd think about it. The breeder showed me pictures of the pups, one of them dashing around with a piece of sock in her mouth and her head up high as if she owned the world, while all the others just lolled. That was Vita, and she really was the pick of the litter.

I seem always to present Vita as the perfect dog, and in many ways she is. At 55 pounds she is small for a Labrador, but she makes up for it with tremendous drive and an IQ in the Mensa range—and she is ideal for the Super Cub I had for years. A Cub is a small, narrow plane with tandem seating. I had a takeoff prop on it so I could get into and out of small places while duck-hunting. If I wanted to take a friend, Vita was small enough to sit behind the passenger seat and not destroy my weight and balance, even with our guns, ammunition, decoys, blinds and, hopefully, lots of birds on the way home. If I had an especially heavy passenger or too many birds, or the wind was wrong for takeoff after hunting, I would leave the passenger on the flats and fly Vita and all the gear home, then after refueling return for the passenger. (I'd let the castaway keep his shotgun while I was gone.)

But Vita isn't entirely perfect. I frequently take her for long walks in an abandoned gravel pit near my home. It is ideal for its location and for the puddles that draw migratory birds in the fall, leaving wonderful smells for bird dogs. Willows thrive there, and moose like to browse. One fall day as we walked I congratulated myself on having such an industrious hunting dog. Vita hunted every bit of cover, and I knew there was no way she could ever miss a single bird anywhere. We finally ambled on home, and she ran whining to the door to be let in. "What's the rush," I wondered, but let her in while I checked the mailbox.

When I opened the door I saw that Vita was perfect, all right. She was perfectly awful. She had vomited a huge pile of moose poop onto the entry rug. It wasn't birds she was hunting, but moose poop. Good grief! I cleaned most of it up, took the rug to the cleaner, and let them know what had soiled it so they had the best chance of getting the remainder out of the rug.

The day I returned to pick it up I gave my name to the woman in charge and asked for the rug. Her eyes were wide as she asked, "How did the moose get into your house?"

Atka, Nov. 12, 2004

Dear June,

Greetings from the Aleutians! I intended to write you after I took a course in the new and very sophisticated Telemed equipment. It will dramatically change health care in the Bush and I am very excited about it. I can instantly send EKG's to the hospital in Anchorage, and they have a terrific digital camera with all sorts of attachments so I can send really accurate pictures of the skin lesions, ear drums, tonsils, teeth, cervices—anything. Then I fill out a history form and the specialist responds. It costs over $1,400 round trip to travel here from Anchorage, and the weather is always unpredictable. How marvelous to send pictures instead of a patient! I feel blest to have been active in the Bush all these years and to see medicine advance so rapidly in my life span. When I started, the women had never had Pap smears, and now a minimally trained health aide can do an excellent job. Now if they can just figure out how to do orthopedics!

I was supposed to come out here Tuesday, and after we sat at the airport for four hours they decided to try. I was ready to trudge aboard when a friend with a cell phone told me that she had called Dutch and it was still below minimums there and she wasn't going to fly all the way out there just to fly back (four hours each way). I pulled my luggage and went home. Sure was glad, because they didn't make it and had to spend the night in Cold Bay.

I'm telling you all this so you will understand the difficulties in sending a patient to town.

Repeated the whole process on Wednesday. Because I'm going for a month I have a cooler with frozen food; a large box of canned goods and some fresh foods, bread, rice, pudding mix, etc.; suitcase for clothes; box for boots and hiking gear; box for books and music tapes; a shotgun to hunt birds; and a dog crate for my Labrador, with a bag of food taped to the top. It's not like you just take your laptop and go.

So we're off, almost on time. Full load—two days worth of passengers. Nice ride since I've remembered to wear wool socks and insulated snow boots. The floor on those commuter planes is freezing.

Finally it's time to let down into Dutch, and that's when the fun starts. Lots of turbulence through the clouds, and then we are only a hundred feet above the waves with no sign of anything familiar. I see the passengers across the aisle searching as well. "Any sign of Eider Point?" "Can you see Hog Island?" The wheels are down and we are in slow flight with full flaps when a cliff appears out of the clouds and the pilot retracts the wheels and gives it full power as he makes an exciting 180-degree climbing turn. Our faces are white, but then we break out into the clear—and now I see we are going to make the dreaded circular approach, where you skim the mountains behind the town on one wing and then at *less* then a hundred feet make a left pylon turn around the aerial on Standard Oil Hill and plop it down, hopefully on the runway and not in the bay. Then quickly reverse engines so you don't run off the other end of the runway, which has been shortened every year by the storm action of the sea. We make it, but since they had so many passengers there was no

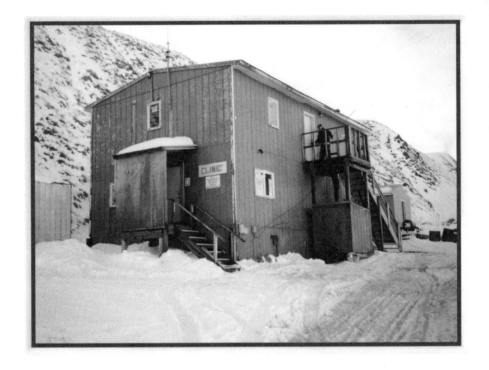

THE ATKA CLINIC *occupied the entire first floor
of a building shared with city government.*

room for luggage. They did bring my dog. You see why I tape the food to her kennel—where she goes, it goes. The luggage is promised for 4 o'clock, then 5, and finally at 6:30 it arrives —all of it, which doesn't always happen. They have canceled the flight to Atka, another two hours away, so we hole up at the Grand Aleutian.

PenAir has told us not to bother even calling about the flight to Atka until 11 or 11:30 a.m., so in the morning I take the dog for a walk. I visit my old haunts, check to see if the museum is open, and wander back to my room about 10, in time to receive a frantic call from a fellow passenger at the airport who says they are loading the plane to Atka, ready for takeoff, and where am I? It isn't easy, but with hotel help I gather my frozen food from their freezer, pile my boxes and bags on a cart, and they get us out there OK. Of course, when I run panting up to the counter the agent says, "Don't rush, we're on weather hold for Atka." At least I get to see old friends from Nikolski who are also on weather hold (but get to fly in the old blue bathtub of the Grumman Goose, my favorite aircraft).

Now we're in Atka. We made it in OK, my dog just behind me in her kennel, and I am housed in "quarters" just above the clinic, where everything is familiar. The handle to the refrigerator door is still missing, the piece of plasterboard I use to hold jigsaw puzzles is still behind the bedroom door, as is the window screen for keeping the healthy rat population out. I'll change *that* today! The little tape player is still on the table, and I brought all of the wonderful tapes a friend made for me. I store all of my gear and food and settle in. I learn not to start thinking immediately about whether I will get out on time.

So you see how valuable Telemed is. Think of that sick patient who must be accompanied, or someone sitting in a dimly lit airport with an ill child for hours on end.

HOORAH for Telemed!

Nancy

Nikolski, spring 2004

Dear Linda,

This box is for the 8-year-old Linda, so please keep your 60-year-old nose out of it. It is for her because I don't think she had many people bringing her the wonders of this beautiful world. Please be kind to her as you would be to your granddaughter, Sophie. Let her have gifts and joy.

Glass balls are rare now, but this day I awoke knowing I would find one for her. I wasn't even surprised when I was joined by dozens of my totem foxes. I knew they would lead me to one. I have often been with foxes but never so many—sleeping on the hillside, curled on the sand in the sun—just blinking as I walked by—and always three accompanying me although they had a changing of the guard. As one dropped off another would join—you will understand.

And then when I finally reached Okee Point past the tip of Anangula Island across the bay, there it was peeping out at me from under a log. What joy—what bliss—I sang to the foxes, I sang to God and I sang to you. Twas wondrous.

The shells are just ones I liked and picked up on the beach. Fragile sea urchin in the paper. If shells aren't your thing, they are great crunched in the garden or on a walk.

—N.

Announcement

I'm going to tell the whole world
you slept with me.
Won't add that you only nodded off
next to me in church.
What impious dreams I had
of you snoring gently in my arms,
the two of us safe together.

Anticipation

Will you stay for breakfast?

We'll have pancakes with berries big as grapes,
flown home by Super Cub rising and falling
toward you on the burbling air.
I will laugh at your lavender lips closing
round the risen batter loaded with fruit,
dripping with the sweetness of syrup,

What a feast we will have.

Sine Te

Sine te—I write it in the sand
of this solitary beach,
couched in Latin lest some mermaid
steal my message and deliver it to you.

Sine te—in the sand so the waves
will erase it and leave me free.

A Rare Thing

Raven's breath,
he said in awe.
How many have
seen the breath of a raven,
white plume rising in icy air
above blackest bird?
A gift, he said.

Gentle man.
How many have
seen one who would notice?

Letters from St. Paul

Nov. 16, 2005 — Wednesday.

Dear Sue,

The wind is howling outside. The furnace refuses to respond. I have kept the ink from freezing by turning the oven on and opening the door. It has been quite an arrival. The plane left on time out of Anchorage on Sunday about 6 p.m. (APIA forgot to give me unlimited baggage so I had to pay $50 extra for my cooler, or maybe for the box with all my books and the eight tapes to *A Jewel in the Crown*. Oh, well, easy flight, and I dined on the Subway sandwich the stewardess gave me.) I got in about 10 p.m., but there was no one to greet me or get me to the condo (the really nice 3-bedroom one to which I can invite guests). I finally spotted Fred, the computer guy, who went out in the parking lot and found the clinic van with the keys tucked into the visor. He told me he had been booked into the condo and I was to stay in one of the clinic quarters. He drove me and his condo buddies to town but found the keys didn't fit the door to quarters. We finally got into the clinic and by going through the meeting room and a labyrinth of halls and stairs broke out into my quarters. It was like stepping into a deep freeze. The furnace had not been alerted to my arrival.

Dear Fred said he would sleep on a couch in the condo and I could have his bed, but I thought I could manage at the clinic. I went to the bathroom, and when I flushed the toilet overflowed. Auspicious beginning. At that point Ben and

Chris, the two health aides, showed up. Ben went down to light the furnace while I plugged in electric heaters and Chris mopped up the mess in the bathroom.

A long time ago you gave me a beanbag to put in the microwave and use as a hot pad. Fortunately I had packed it, so I used it to preheat the bed. The mattress was very cold, but with the beanbag and four blankets I slept very well—only one wandering trip in the night to find another bathroom. I was relieved at the thought of sleeping in since I didn't have to be at work until 10 a.m.

Hah! Phone screeching at 7 a.m.—the boys had an upper GI bleeder coming in. At least it was warm in the clinic. No IV Ritidine (which I love) and the patient's Hgb. is falling. Called ANMC and got a doctor who said to use gastric lavage before we called medivac. We got a line in and rounded up what would do for a nasal/gastric (NG) tube. It was huge and stiff because it had two channels instead of the normal one, but I got it down his nose and managed to hit the esophagus instead of his trachea. We washed him out with normal saline and wonder of wonders, no clots broke loose to let gallons out, and the fluid finally came back clear! I was delighted. I gave him oral Ritidine and Valium for his upcoming alcohol withdrawal symptoms and sent him home—alcohol gastritis instead of bleeding peptic ulcer or esophageal varices.

Our boss, Jessica, made the boys trade apartments with me. Actually, they were to have done so before I arrived but "hadn't gotten around to it." So at least I now have a functioning toilet. (Except when the wind exceeds 45 knots and the Venturi effect on the vent pipe sucks all the water out of the bowl. I tell people that this is the only place I know of with tides in the toilet.)

I collapsed into bed Monday night after a very busy day plus a walk after work to visit the seals. Still a lot of pups out on the point. I love to see them and their moms. There was a gorgeous full moon.

And then came Tuesday. First an 80-year-old man with hip fracture. Chris took the call and did the home visit, saying he thought it was just a dislocation. In an 80-year-old? I don't think so. I got the ambulance to bring him in and took an x-ray. He had a nasty fracture of the upper femur. (His whole family came to sit with him—I liked that.) Another gent came in with chest pain radiating bilaterally and a history of infarction in 1998.

Meanwhile, Alaska Native Medical Center has a new pharmacist who is so anal it is startling. She won't accept English on an Rx, only Latin. Of course the aides are writing the refills and they don't know Latin. They clearly say understandable things like one pill 2X a day. However this twit keeps calling to say she can't fill a "non-legal" prescription that doesn't say "bid" instead of 2X a day. I think she will have a mental breakdown if she continues to work there. . . .

I slept like a log last night. Today has been a comparative breeze. I had only one man I am worried about. He had a temp of 102 and vomiting with a sore throat. Positive strep test so I gave penicillin. I hope he doesn't have meningitis. Neck OK when I saw him.

Dinner time. More later, maybe.

Love,

Nancy

Feb. 19, 2006.

Dear Art,

I am being so "good" out here that I stink. I get up early and spend at least two hours on poetry, trying to "clean the rust out of my pipes." I do an hour of yoga after work, and the weather determines the length of the daily hike I take. You see why this seems like a retreat to me. The computer and TV are here but not yet hooked up. There is only one radio station, which broadcasts the local basketball games. At present I am the only one in itinerant quarters in the new clinic. Chaos reigns since the staff is still in the process of moving from the old TB hospital on the hill that used to be my "home."

The first noon here I was all alone; everyone else had gone home to lunch. The janitor came and got me for a woman who was "crying." I'm glad I was here because she had overdosed on her insulin and her blood glucose was 18! (70 is low normal.) Where to find the glucagon in all this mess? I dashed to the pharmacy and was discouraged by the shelf after shelf of STUFF—and then I saw the familiar bright orange packets "ready to go." I managed to get it into her before she seized, and all was well.

I expect this tour to go well—the first night here the foxes greeted me, barking outside my window until I fell asleep. I suppose we see what we want in life.

Love,
Nancy

Feb. 26, 2006.

Dear Bruce and Sandy,

I'm having a very exciting time out here. I went to the basketball games in the gym last night and watched the high school girls beat the village women (unmercifully). I thought I should have brought oxygen and a good medical kit when I saw all those overweight diabetics running around. Then the boys' game began about 9 p.m. Admission was $2, and an entire dinner of chicken plate, soda, popcorn or ice cream was also available. The boys played the Wasilla Christian School—the latter were on the average one foot or so taller. Much hooting and stamping of feet. I'm on call so had to leave to take care of a man who had abdominal pain, intractable vomiting and diarrhea. He had managed to keep down six to eight (his count—probably more) beers, however. I diagnosed it as alcoholic gastritis, so gave him ranitidine and called a "keeper" to keep him off beer and to dole out Librium for his withdrawal. Back to the game, and the "Sea Parrots," who had been ahead when I left, were now trailing, not for want of an enthusiastic crowd.

I was amazed when a woman, the temporary English teacher, sat next to me and called me Nancy. I finally realized she was my first poetry teacher at UAA. I just never know whom I will meet out here. I'm going to try to have her over for dinner this week. She is very nice, and funny as well. I bet the kids love her. She sure likes them.

Then I had to go see a little boy who had poked his eyeball with a toothpick. It was swollen shut and a big mess. I will see him again today and if he's not better send him out on tonight's plane.

The last one I saw was an 82-year-old diabetic with an insulin reaction, so I didn't get to see the end of the game. The Sea Parrots probably lost. I love the name. Not the feisty, tough "Beach Masters," not the "Polar Bears," but the "Sea Parrots." See why I like it out here?

My Achilles tendon is acting up again so I haven't gone on as many walks as usual. In addition, the clinic has been extremely busy. I am expected to supervise and teach three village aides on all the patients they see as well as take care of my own patients. I run out of steam by 6 o'clock, which is when I usually get done. I love teaching, especially since there is one woman here who really wants to learn. She is like a sponge, sopping up every scrap of information she comes across. She will become a PA, I am sure, and under different circumstances would have been an M.D. She will be at UAF for one year starting next fall. I don't want to come here when she is gone—well, maybe the other two aides will be more advanced by then.

We are in the new clinic now and not the old TB hospital. It is very fancy and must have cost a fortune, but I can't get a simple CBC (complete blood count) or even a hemoglobin. I am going to the top brass on that one. They do have a good x-ray machine, but no one knows how to use it. I think things will be better after they get the moving done. Half the stuff is still in the old building.

The dentist and two assistants are here in itinerant quarters with me. They really work hard. They start promptly at 8 a.m. and work straight through until 9 or 9:30 p.m. every day for two weeks. Because this is Sunday, they are quitting early—at 7:30—and have invited me to dinner. I will cook so it will be ready when they get finished. I also went to the unique liquor store (only wine and beer). The entrance is from an alley behind an old warehouse where I pick my way through discarded 5-gallon buckets, old bicycle parts and other garbage to the inner door. I got a bottle of wine to have with dinner. When I got home I realized there was no corkscrew anywhere. I searched the clinic, went back to the old one and looked through drawers there. Finally figured that this guy was a dentist and could drill the cork out if need be. And he may have to.

     Love,

     Mom

Atka

Nov. 12, 2006—*Sunday.*

I was amazed that I left Anchorage on time last week
(after paying $160 excess baggage for Vita, my gun, extra
books and groceries), but in Dutch the airline found a mechanical problem on the Navajo so the Atka flight was canceled. I
got a room at the Grand Aleutian and called to see if the clinic
needed me. It was a vacation day for them. Made arrangements with Susan, for whom I had worked previously, to meet
on Saturday morning for dog walking—she has a male lab.
She hadn't found the hot spring so we set off in search of that.
We drove out to Summer Bay in her clinic car and found the
hot spring (I hadn't been there since 1995 but remembered
where it was), and the dogs had a ball. I got back in time to
catch my flight to Atka and watched *all* my bags being loaded.
I think that is a first. I remember one time in Nikolski when
the airline kept one box of groceries the entire two weeks and
I picked them up on my way home.

Once here I had the usual quick lowdown on clinic matters from Irene, the woman I am replacing, as she boarded the
plane to return to Dutch. I had a van to drive! Oh, joy! I
could explore farther from home. I am to stay in the new
clinic housing and not upstairs in the funky quarters above
the clinic with its two bedrooms and a bath. Too bad. I am so
accustomed to no view, where to find the piece of sheetrock
for my jigsaw puzzle, how to prop the window open at night,

recognizing the grunts and snorts of the old refrigerator, and having no walk to work, which makes lunch a breeze. When I walked into this house with three bedrooms and a large kitchen/living room, I hated it. Whoever lived here has really trashed it. I see holes in all the doors, locks broken, one bedroom stuffed with junk—mattresses, frames, etc. All the lights are hanging by wires, most bulbs are missing, and mold is an inch thick in the bathroom. I could have cried.

The van had a flat tire and because it was Sunday, I couldn't rent a 4-wheeler. I took the radio and Vita for a long walk over to the Bering Sea side just to get out of here. I was still feeling depressed when I got back. After pouting for 24 hours, I noticed that Irene had left me a big pot of delicious reindeer stew. I called Millie about the tire. She came over with a pump and we had tea and cookies while the pump filled the tire. Then the neighbors next door brought a plate of goodies (fried Spam and salmon cakes). They are so kind to me out here and treat me like one of them. I realized I had sure been an ass—I have what is really important. Place seems OK to me now. I should sleep better tonight. With the window open I can hear the surf on the beach. The sound dispels the violence I feel in this house. Oh, and Millie told me where the ptarmigan hang out.

The Hot Spring

A smiling sybarite am I
since at last I found
the hot spring in the tundra.
My hot tub in the grass—
all else snowbound.

A smiling sybarite am I.
A swan in golden feathers
on a satin pond.
Neck extended, black eyes aglow,
I flow through the mist as though
God drew me.

A smiling sybarite am I.
A trout in mountain stream
washing my scales in delicious dance
as each molecule of wetness
trickles down my flank.

A smiling sybarite am I.
A postulate for orders
in my baptismal bath.
I sing God's praise in firm new voice
so that the fox can hear.

Dutch Harbor

Jan. 4, 2007 — Thursday.

THIS TRIP I AM TO REPLACE ANNETTE, the PA at the Oonalaska Wellness Center (operated by APIA), while she goes out for more training. I have Vita with me, and Annette needs someone to care for her dog and two cats, so I will stay in her house and not have to live in the hotel for weeks with a dog. But what a tour so far!

PenAir was an hour late out of Anchorage on the 30th of December. It flew in to Cold Bay to refuel and then on to Dutch. We were in a holding pattern while an earlier plane attempted unsuccessfully to land, and then it was our turn. Severe low-level wind shear, so the plane was all over the sky as we passed Eider Point and then Hog Island on final approach. It was wild over the runway, and I wanted him to go around! Go around! But he stuck it on and slapped the brakes on so we didn't go off the other end of the runway into the bay. Whew! We were the only ones to make it in.

Annette was there to meet me. Then it socked in and she couldn't get out for three days. I holed up in the Grand Aleutian and even found a place to run Vita. The snow was so deep that I had to find plowed but seldom used roads. From the hotel I went over behind Eagle Grocery and then to the mouth of Margaret Bay, where a construction company has quarters.

1-6-07

SATURDAY—I AM at Annette's house now. Yesterday when I got up I opened the door to let the dogs out and found a drift higher than my head. And where was the shovel? In the back seat of the car, of course. I crawled up and out and although I could get to the car, the doors were frozen shut. I tried all four to no avail and then got really mad and managed to get the right rear door open. I kicked the other doors open from the inside. Holding the latch open while kicking was as good as any yoga but perhaps not as tranquil. I got the shovel and dug the house door open and let the dogs out while I cleared the driveway. Snow was so high I could barely throw it up to the top of the berm. I was only a little late to work, where the aide told me to spray oil on the rubber door seals to keep them from freezing. Of course I locked the door to the duplex when I went to work and it was frozen when I came home. I feel like a real cheechako.

Today is Saturday, the start of a three-day weekend (Russian Christmas), so I am doing a load of wash and will try to clean house. Then I will take the dogs for a real walk and get some #8 screws from True Value to reattach the bathroom door. I have given up on the landlord. The door had previously been held on by only one ¾-inch screw. At least the heat is back on. It was out while Annette was here. Of course, snow is falling again, so I will shovel the drive and hope the wind doesn't blow it all back.

Work at the clinic has gone well, thanks to Irene, the village health aide, and Chris, who works at the front desk. The most fascinating case was a 50-year-old woman who had had a bilateral mastectomy and is being prepped for augmentation. There were beautiful instructions from the Anchorage surgeon. Each week we inject about 60 cubic centimeters of normal saline with Ancef into the plastic container under her skin. This has a port located by a magnet. Her last injection will be next week. The physician is making room for her new breasts by enlarging the space a little at a time.

Another interesting case is a 40-year-old man with a past history of alcohol and drug abuse. He also has dementia secondary to carbon monoxide poisoning, which occurred after a "wrestling match" while drinking with a friend. The exhaust on his kerosene heater dislodged, and in his stupor he just passed out and was not found until the next day. His headaches have increased recently, and lo and behold, his serology came back positive for syphilis.

It is light out now so I will get on with the day.

· ·

Later—9 p.m. I got #10 screws and fixed the bathroom door. I thought I could walk the dogs out past True Value, where I bought the screws, but the roads were being plowed so I headed up Captain's Bay and parked at the top of the hill and walked a couple of miles, part of it in deep snow. A whiteout occurred suddenly and I couldn't see two feet. Because Vita is black she showed up best in trying to find our way. I could barely see our tracks in the snow before they drifted in. I was glad to get back to the car.

I'm knitting a prayer shawl for each of my kids to have when I die, and I just finished the blue one. Now I only have to put the fringe on it. Unalaska seems the right place to finish it—the blue always makes me think of both the water and the shade of blue I see in the sky here. It is a very nice day.

1-8-07, Russian Orthodox Christmas.

MONDAY—THE ICICLES AT THE window are dripping so the predicted warmth has arrived. Strange to look out and not see it snowing. Clinic closed so I am changing the bed linens, cleaning (evermore) and getting ready to take the dogs for a good run. I will grocery shop on my way home and take letters to the post office to mail.

I thought I was in the soup last night. A phone call came about a young man who, 15 minutes after eating, noted his tongue swelling and was having difficulty breathing. I leapt out of bed trying to remember where the epinephrine was stored in the clinic because this sounded like anaphylaxis, which can kill in minutes. I worried on my way in whether I should have called the Iliuliuk Clinic in advance for backup. It has much more sophisticated technology than in our little clinic. When I saw him I couldn't believe he was the same patient who had called. He was so normal—even had a slow pulse. It was a panic attack that he had. Was I ever relieved, and glad I hadn't called the other clinic.

· ·

LATER: I WENT TO TAKE THE DOGS OUT but saw a patient at the office on the way. After that I went on up to the trail leading up the back side of Pyramid Peak. The dogs and I walked a mile or so and then back, looking for a place to train Vita. I finally drove out to the garbage dump where the city crew was shoving snow into the bay. I saw a big cleared area and asked the D-8 Cat driver if I could train away from where he was working. I set up first a double and then a triple blind. Vita handled very well. The driver of a snow truck saw her and asked if I could teach his dog to do that. "She's yellow and dumb as a stick," he said. I told him it took a lot of time. Nice to be appreciated and not run off.

I stopped to mail letters and my cell phone rang so I had to go back to the office. Then I made an unsuccessful trip to the grocery for a newspaper. I stopped at the library to see Cora and asked her to dinner. This is a difficult time for her. Milt died suddenly in their home a short time ago. He had had multiple medical problems. Cora works until 9 p.m. most days but has Wednesday and Thursday off, so I will try to see what we can arrange.

1-9-07

TUESDAY—A NEW day with winds to 30 knots and pouring rain. The slush is a sight to behold. I wallowed to work OK but got stuck in the drive this noon. Heavy shoveling. The clinic is closed this afternoon because of weather. The winds increased to 80 knots and rain persisted. I dashed home and got the dogs for a walk before it got worse. By getting used to all this wind Vita ought to be a whiz on crosswind blinds. I had leftover stew for dinner and am having cocoa while listening to David Harding play viola on the "Goldberg Variations." Nice balance to knee-high slush outside. I did my best on shoveling but it is just too much. I did get my car off the street, which was no mean accomplishment. Bed looks very appealing.

1-14-07

SUNDAY—I AM WENDING my way through breakfast, Vita asleep next to me, Misty staring out the window, Marco Polo asleep on my bed, and Molly, Annette's dog, in the corner. Bears beating the Seahawks on mute TV. It was a beautiful day Friday so I convinced Abi to slide down the hill and come to dinner. Lively as usual. President Bush, in his Wednesday speech, said he intends to invade Iran and Syria. The guy is bonkers.

Jerah's friend David has gone home. It will be a loss to the town if Jerah leaves, too. He is an excellent poet and very active in the arts here. Our dinner was interrupted by tsunami warnings. The tsunami was to reach Shemya at 9:30 p.m. (it was 9 p.m. then) and here around 11:30. This house is on Standard Oil Hill, which is a "to go to" place, so I relaxed. The warning got called off later.

I drove on a heavy crust of snow out Captain's Bay Road with the dogs and got some great marks and blinds in for Vita. She was much more content last night. Looks like I can do it again today. Tomorrow is Martin Luther King Day, so the clinic is closed. I like three-day weekends, although this is the last.

I am almost through one skein of yarn on the last prayer shawl. Naturally I haven't fixed the pocket on my corduroy trousers, and there is an iron here so I have no excuse.

Later: The codeine addict I thought I had gotten rid of (by not giving her more than eight at a time) called and now wants to come back for care. Of course she said she needed T 4s, which are Tylenol with 60 mg of codeine. I gave her only eight T 3s, which have only 30 mg of codeine, and she will see Dr. Cotten on Tuesday to try to get more. I'm all in favor of a conference with the clinic doctors downstairs so she doesn't manipulate her way between the two clinics.

Out with the dogs and I got that little Mazda up and down the hills clear to the water tank. I set up a series of marks for Vita, all of which she nailed. Molly went with me, but Vita could get to the marks first even though she was 150 yards farther away. These were just "fun" marks for exercise, and Vita really went all out to be first there. Then I set up three really good blinds around the marks. They were all uphill, with varied terrain and exposed brush and crusted snow with ptarmigan scent. The first was only 100 yards or so; the second one was right over the mark, then the third was at least 250 yards and up a really steep side hill. She took every cast on all three of them.

I am going to Abi's for dinner tonight. Found a pomegranate to have with Abi's applesauce dessert. She has a DVD she wants me to watch after dinner. I'll probably fall asleep after my mountain climbing on that glazed snow crust with the dogs. I was up quite high, and coming down is always trickier than ascending. I was inching down when I finally decided what the heck, this is taking all day and I'm sure to slip and fall somewhere, so I just lay down on my back and shot down to the road. Was Vita ever excited! Molly couldn't keep up. Nice afternoon. It disturbs me that while I see grownups out walking, I haven't seen any kids. How can they stay in when it is so gorgeous?

. .

Gift

Midnight.

The cut crystal light

of the round steely moon skitters

across the glazed surface of the lake.

Music of blade on ice floats on frozen air.

The moon falls deep

among the weeds and fishes.

I glide through clouds, scattering

stars in twice reflected light,

through schools of liquid motion, feeling

scales against my cheeks,

fins through my hair.

Breaching the weeds I skim

unfettered among distant worlds, whirl

through beckoning spirals and nebulas,

lose myself in the vastness and

for this brief moment

am home.

WELL, SO LONG TO SUDOKU! I HAVE returned from dinner with Abi with Aldous Huxley's *The Devils of Loudun*, a three-hour video version of Peter Brook's *Mahabarata*, and *The Tough Winter*, by Robert Lawson. I also have her snowshoes (with crampon-like edges) and ski poles. It will take me at least an hour to come down from all that stimulation. The pomegranate with the applesauce was divine.

1-15-07

MONDAY—I COULD see the weather was changing this morning so hurried around and got the washing done, put three big sacks of garbage into the car, loaded dogs, and went up Captain's Bay Road again. This time I used Abi's good snowshoes. The wind was howling but I got in a series of good marks and two blinds. I had been drinking tea all morning at home and my bladder was threatening to burst, so I found a sort of gully where it wasn't blowing so hard and, still on snowshoes, hurriedly lowered my pants. What a relief—and then I noticed there was no "yellow snow." How could that be? Lesson No. 1: When peeing in the wind, be sure to either face or back directly into the wind or your pant leg will get soaked. Oh, well, I felt better. I went to the dump and found it closed for Martin Luther King Day. Drat! The whole car stunk from the garbage, so I drove over to East Point, where I stayed the last time I was in town, and dumped all the sacks into the dumpster there.

I proceeded home and made a swell lunch of mango, pear and more of that pomegranate, with cottage cheese and yogurt. Hadn't been home long when the wind got worse, and now it is blowing snow and rain against the windows. The dogs are tired and content and so am I, snugly drinking hot chocolate. I am so glad I went early!

1-21-07

SUNDAY—I HAVE been so busy there has been no time to write. I will just hit the high spots. After the big storm, I took the dogs back out Captain's Bay Road. It was pretty slushy so I pulled in to the first Y and ran the dogs from there. No train-ing, just running. I was about to go home when my cell phone rang—a patient needing to be seen. I told her I was near and would meet her at the clinic in 10 minutes. Hah!—I was stuck in the slush and no amount of backward and forward effort was successful. I got the shovel out and dug and dug and as I was doing that I heard, "Would you like me to give you a push?' This is very off the beaten path and I seldom see any-one up there in this weather. It was a hiker "just out for a walk." With him pushing I got out fine. It made me feel good, and I was only a little late at the clinic doling out Nicoderm for a patient whose daughter said she was "freaking out."

Cora came to dinner Thursday night. I had made crab bisque but everything was late because Marco Polo, Annette's cat, was dying before my eyes. Poor thing. He was the one of her pets I liked the best. He had lost the use of his back legs so couldn't get into the pot box. I made him a "low-rise," but he couldn't do that, either, so peed on the rug, vomited and refused all food. He hid in the pantry. I ached for him. I called Annette and got permission to have him put down, which they do at the police station here. The police will not release the body to the owner because it is loaded with sodium lumi-nal, a sedative, and people bury too shallow so the eagles and foxes dig up the bodies to eat and then die of the sodium luminal. The officer explained that they have a special place for pets at the dump and they bury them very deep. Annette couldn't stand to have him buried "in the dump," so I talked the officer into letting me have the body if I promised cremation. He was very nice. I ran home, got poor Marco and took him down. He was as relaxed as my old lab, Amy, when I had to put her down. He seemed just glad to have it over. I rushed back to work, finished, and then picked up the dogs and called Cora, who wanted to go on our walk with us. We all walked up the Pyramid Peak trail as far as the pump house. Cora was glad to get out.

I drove her home for dinner, which was most pleasant. I had gotten a bottle of what we call "the Janitor's Wine." The janitor at the clinic is part of a wine-growing family in California. The liquor stores in Dutch carry the Borrego label, with a very good pinot grigio. When the time came to pour, I discovered there was no corkscrew in the house—shades of St. Paul when I treated the dental crew to a bottle and they had to drill the cork out. "Why not put a screw in the cork and pull it out by that?" Cora asked. I had some screws left from fixing the bathroom door so I put one in and used pliers to pull the cork—*bon appetit*! We had a very good time. I think it was good for her to get out of the house where Milt died.

I took her home after dinner and picked Marco Polo up at the police station on my way home. I can't mail a dead cat so I will keep his body in the freezer here and take him to Anchorage as luggage. He will go to the crematorium where Annette has made arrangements. I found the entire episode drained me emotionally. Even in this short time I could see what a great cat he was—like my old Fosdick, just special.

My birthday was yesterday. I slept in until 8 and it was wonderful. I drank tea and read the last of my hoarded Anchorage newspapers. I was still tired so puttered, then went to the office to see a couple of patients and check my e-mail. It was nice to get birthday greetings there.

I had decided to go to the annual meeting of the Aleutian Arts Council at the Grand Aleutian Hotel at 7 p.m. It was to be a brief meeting, silent auction of donated art, live auction, dinner, a free T-shirt to new members, and music for dancing by the "Ballyhooters." That is what got me—the Ballyhooters! I tore home to change clothes and discovered that the inner door was locked. Annette had warned me never to lock it because there was no key. It had been taped so it wouldn't lock, and I had had no problem. Rats! So there I was, next to the washer and dryer and the dog food, in the entryway. I jiggled and pounded to no avail. Then I noticed the hinge pins were on my side of the door and a screwdriver was on the shelf. I pulled the pins and, using a file to hold the bottom of the door off the floor, pulled it from the hinge and got in. The secret was that the little knob that has to be turned, on most locks, in this case only needs to be depressed. If it were mine I would change that for an un-lockable pantry door latch.

I changed very fast and went to the meeting, which was great fun. Jerah was the MC. I ended up at a table with the Iliuliuk clinic docs and a temporary teacher from Montana, whom I immediately liked. I looked at the arts and crafts, not expecting much, but did see a set of tea towels with puffins on them and one mono-print that fascinated me. I tried for the towels on the dollar bid where everyone keeps putting dollars in a bucket until the bell rings and whoever is putting a dollar in at that moment gets the item. I tried unsuccessfully to con the winner out of one of the three in the set. The food was excellent. The last art piece to go was a painting by Caroline Reed of Abi in her skiff, which reminded me of that wonderful trip. Heidi Bains, the M.D. from the Iliuliuk Clinic, bought it. I ended up with a print I liked and still like today. It is by Laresa Syverson, a Native woman who has the traditional tattoos. She wasn't there, but I would like to meet her. The Ballyhooters were good, with guitars, keyboard, sax and tympani. I happily went home and had just gotten there when I was asked to make a house call on a dying woman. Irene, the health aide, went with me. Bless her. Hospice would be nice here. Kath from the Wellness Center was there, too.

What I haven't mentioned about the day is the beautiful "sky displays." It was like watching the weather station satellite views on fast-forward. One minute it was clear, brilliant light and the next, deep blue velvet followed by snow. I saw photographers out trying to catch it and I did, too, but know mine can't begin to show what I saw. All in all, it was a very good day.

Snowing this morning but it doesn't look serious. I'll wait until noon and dig out for a dog and garbage run and to check e-mail.

1-22-07

MONDAY—ANOTHER shoveling day. At least Dr. Cotten got in, which saved me the nightmare of an infected carpal tunnel surgery. I was happy to work on the botched methotrexate order from pharmacy. Irene's daughter is having us both over for dinner tomorrow, and the next day I will go to Cora's home. It is very nice to have dinner with conversation. I am tired tonight and already in what I call "Departure Mode."

I'm reading the Aldous Huxley book Abi gave me, which is familiar after the Education for Ministry class I took at home. Huxley is quite a switch from the dog training book Clare sent. I'll fix dinner (microwave dinner heated in the regular oven) with green beans. Butterscotch pudding for dessert. And I am still losing weight! Must be the dog walks.

1-24-07

WEDNESDAY—BLIZZARD with blowing snow and winds to 50 mph predicted to increase to 70 mph. Dogs were happy to get home from our walk, and so was I. A busy day with Dr. Cotten here. She is from Halibut Cove near Homer, Alaska, and I know her father, Clem Tillion. I like her very much and she knows the system well; it takes her very little time to make appointments for our patients to see doctors at the hospital in Anchorage when consults are needed. I will not go to Cora's tonight because of the weather. I'll try again tomorrow. I am happy to stay home. Driving is impossible. Visibility is less than two feet in the blowing snow.

1-25-07

TUESDAY—WEATHER is worse today. Clinic and schools are closed, over two feet of snow on our road, and it is still coming down. Wind is about the same. I had to shovel my way out of the house to let the dogs out. Dr. Cotten is at the hotel so may be able to get to the clinic to give an antibiotic shot to my sick baby. I think he will survive without it but will do better with it. Weather is supposed to last until six this evening. With this wind there is no way the crews can keep roads open. I may get a new pocket sewn in my cords after all.

. .

Later: I did it! The pocket is in! And there are worse things than sitting inside a snug house during a blizzard listening to Serkin and Rostropovich play the Brahms cello sonatas.

St. Paul

May 6, 2007—Sunday.

IT HAS BEEN A ROUGH COUPLE OF DAYS. I got called out of the basketball game to make a house call to see a woman in her fifties who weighs over 250 pounds, is diabetic, has severe chronic obstructive pulmonary disease (COPD) but still smokes. She was having trouble breathing and was very agitated and uncooperative—signs of low oxygen. She refused to come to the clinic. She had just gotten back from Anchorage where they had only done a mammogram. She is on constant oxygen at 3 L per minute and has Albuterol nebulizers. She told me she was just tired and couldn't sleep. Her O_2 Sats were surprisingly OK at 98, and her respiratory rate was in the low twenties. I couldn't hear anything in her lungs so I called ER in Anchorage and they agreed with me to just give 1 mg of Ativan. I went back to the house to give it to her, taking only one dose because I didn't want anyone to give her more after I left.

I called again on Saturday and went over—it was about 10 a.m. She was worse, with increased respiratory rate and decreased O_2 Sats, so I said, "I'm calling medivac." Of course, she had a fit. I upped her O_2 on her home O_2 concentrator to 5, which is the maximum, and her Sat rose, but I still didn't like it. I called ER again and they set up medivac. Of course it was snowing, and I didn't think the plane would get in.

Meanwhile I got the EMT's to bring her to the clinic. When she got here her Sats were 60! I got a combo mask and gave 6 L O2 plus Albuterol nebulizer. I had already given her 60 mg of prednisone at home. By this time she was somnolent and the EMT's and I had to tie her onto the chair so she wouldn't fall off. I knew we would never get her up. Medivac finally arrived. She left, but she died around noon today. At least she kissed her mom and said, "I love you," as they took her to the ambulance for the plane.

This kind of case makes me both very sad and angry. I wonder what happened to make her so self-destructive, with excessive weight gain plus the smoking to the point of pulmonary failure. I am not angry with her but with life that did something insurmountable to her. I am not a Pollyanna, but I do care.

Jan. 15, 2008 — Tuesday.

I CAME OUT NONSTOP ON DECEMBER 27 to beautiful weather with new snow, sunshine and no wind. I felt I was on the wrong island. I knew to soak it up and store it for when winter hit. I walked 4 to 8 miles on the beaches almost every day. I am concerned about my foxes. I see tracks but haven't seen a fox, so I take scraps out to put near den sites I know from previous times. I even bought hot dogs to help them out. Hope they got them before the seagulls did.

I am alone in quarters here for a change. The gushing water in the pipes is the same as ever. Sleeping under a waterfall is never easy, even with my hearing aids out.

Things went well the first two weeks of this trip, but I went on first call last Friday and the sky fell in. Winter hit with winds greater than 75 mph, blowing snow. The accidents began. One 10-year-old was sledding and hit a barrier. She punctured her lip through to include her gum. She was great—held really still while I sewed. Then came croup, asthma, frozen fingers, migraines, a hernia, etc, etc, etc.

In another sledding accident today, one girl sprained an ankle and the other one had a contusion and deep laceration to her forehead from her titanium eyeglasses, which hit an artery as well as fracturing the outer layer of her cranium. She also had a fracture of her leg bone (femur) with a dislocated hip. I tried to medivac but the weather was too bad—the plane tried from Dutch but had to turn back. I finally got the Coast Guard with their C-130 to try, and they made it about 11:30 p.m. The crews here were frantically clearing drifts from the runway so the plane could land. Crews even backed the plane right up to the hanger to make it possible to load the patient in that miserable weather. At that point the moon came out, the wind stopped and all was well. I was glad because it really was a nasty fracture, and I worry about the head injury.

I fell into bed but got calls for fecal impaction, bleeding from a catheter, and finally one for a gunshot wound to the leg. A fellow cleaned his .45 pistol, drank 10 beers, and decided to "dry fire" it before he put it away. Strangely enough, it wasn't dry fire, and he shot through the upper third of his tibia. He had fierce bleeding, and the x-ray showed a fracture. I tried plain pressure but the bleeding bone wouldn't quit and there was no wax to fill the holes in the bone. I tightened the bandage so it at least slowed down. It is now 6:30 a.m. and flights have been on weather hold since 4 a.m. I don't think he has lost more than 500 cc. Medivac will bring O-neg blood for him. The weather here is pretty good so Anchorage must be holding things up. I feel sorry for the new nurse practitioner. She just wore herself (and me) out with worry, hyperventilating and pacing. I keep trying to tame her hyper state, to no avail. I think I will go brush my teeth.

1-21-08

MONDAY—TODAY I am supposed to go home. The ER is full of patients—a partial amputation of one finger, fractured leg, and possible appendicitis. I helped and cocked an eye to the weather. Four inches of snow fell last night. Fog moved in this morning. Who knows?

Domestic Violence

For years now I have treated patients with black eyes, bruises, broken ribs and noses, and contusions, all of which have been "accidental." Not one patient would admit to being assaulted.

Any treatment I gave addressed only the symptoms and not the cause—domestic violence. That was the equivalent of prescribing cough syrup for pulmonary tuberculosis. It seemed to me that the victims, usually female but sometimes male, felt shame and guilt, which kept them from talking about it.

But there was a kind of breakthrough today. A woman came to talk to me about it. A few nights ago her husband was chasing her around the house with a gun. He was too drunk to navigate the steep stairs, but when she ran up them to use the phone to call the police, he began shooting through the ceiling. She reached the phone, gave her name and told what was happening. The response was, "Oh, you call all the time," followed by a click as the dispatcher hung up on her.

I was astounded, but remembered a film on domestic violence that my friend Diddy Hitchins had lent me. It clearly showed that the violence and the lack of response that so troubled me are not limited to the islands or Alaska or even the United States—and that the victims are not responsible for the violence done against them, rather that such violence is a reflection of a dysfunction in society in general.

I offered to lend the tape to the woman who had come to me and she accepted it with alacrity. I told her I needed to have it back before I left for home, but I was thrilled when she called the next day and asked if she could keep it for a few days more to show to her friends. What an encouraging happening! Now if a new attitude will just spread from village to village.

St. Paul

April 28, 2008—Monday.

I WAS TO DEPART ANCHORAGE AT noon but although the weather was fine, there was a mechanical so I sat until 3, thinking of all the last-minute things I could have been doing at home. In addition, the airport is being remodeled so all the eating places are absent. I noted that the bar was still there. Enough griping.

The eventual trip out was smooth and I got here about 6 p.m. St. Paul airport was a swarm of people. The fifth graders were departing for a tour of California—Disneyland, Knott's Berry Farm, San Diego Zoo. Were they ever happy! It was a delightful melee. Monique, the village aide, was there to meet me. She had come back from a training session in Anchorage to cover because no other aide was here. We went straight to the clinic and got supplies to see Alexay, who has bedsores (very bad ones) and needed a catheter change. It was nice to see him and his wife again. I will check on him again tomorrow because he hasn't had a BM in a week. He is a diabetic with bedsores—sacral ulceration—and an even worse one on his left heel. It is too much for home care, but what to do? I gave a lesson on home care but the sores are probably inevitable. How can that little old woman change his position several times a day? It is never easy for caregivers or loving family members. I can hear my father's voice—he had repeatedly told us that when he died he wanted to be at home surrounded by family. He had had a stroke and was being cared for at home as requested when I went down to the farm to check on him. Mother was under 5 feet tall and of course had trouble moving him. When I arrived and saw the bedsores—plus he had pneumonia—the "doctor" me took over and I insisted he be moved to the hospital. He died three days later and not surrounded by family in his own home. I have always felt guilty of depriving him of his last wishes. There is more to medicine than what you see and hear.

From Alexay's, out to pick up the priest's grandson, who is seven months old and has a low-grade fever and a runny nose. His parents were going to fly to Anchorage tomorrow for the weekend and show him off, but his eardrums were both scarlet and he had 4 plus nasal congestion. I told them I would see him in the morning but am sure he won't be well enough to go.

Finally got to quarters and unpacked, made the bed and heated a microwave dinner. I saw it was already 9:15 p.m. and a long while since I had gotten up at 5:30 this morning.

No fishing or crabbing going on, and the snow is mostly gone, so it ought to be a quiet tour. Nice greetings from lots of people welcoming me back. Makes me feel good.

4-29-08

TUESDAY—QUIET TOUR—hah. Before I could get to bed I had an ER call. A 19-year-old woman had overdosed on Centrum with iron, Flexeril (which causes delusional dementia), Tylenol 3, ibuprofen, and another multiple vitamin. I got all set to pump her stomach out (gastric lavage) but last week in a case of "domestic violence" her nose was broken. I didn't really want to run a tube through her previously damaged nose, so I called ER in Anchorage and got the number for the poison control center in Oregon. They said just charcoal ought to be all right. Monique seemed anxious to take over, and the patient seemed stable, so I gave her the charcoal and went to bed while Monique watched over her.

Time for work and I am already tired.

5-1-08

THURSDAY—THE DAY after the overdose was even busier. A woman came in with strange visual patterns. She had a history of migraines and had a left-sided headache. I was happy to see that we had some Imitrex on the shelf, but a minute after I gave it to her she said her headache was 10 times worse and she turned bright red with a temp of over 100. I called ER in Anchorage and they said to give Compazine, 10 mg IV as well as Benedryl 50 mg IM. Her veins collapsed on just looking for them, plus she weighed over 200 pounds so they were hard to find for the intravenous injection. Monique tried, I tried, but we finally gave up and gave her Compazine 20 mg and Benedryl 50 mg, both intramuscularly. After about 30 minutes she felt fine and her color returned to normal as did her temperature. I was very glad she didn't stop breathing as some Imitrex reactions do.

That exciting occasion was followed by a young man with appendicitis. I finally got him medivac'd out at 5 a.m. (He had a fecolith in his appendix.)

When I got to work yesterday there had been a suicide of a very nice young man. The medical examiner in Anchorage wanted an exam and I am no Kay Scarpetta (a fictional pathologist medical examiner). He wanted vitrious fluid from both eyes and a urine sample as well as blood. This poor man had dressed up for his suicide. He had on well-worn but clean clothes—jeans, t-shirt, flannel shirt, plus a large wooden cross on a thick woven cord around his neck. His glasses were still on. No blood on his clothes—just a few drops in his mouth and the little round hole in his hard palate. It looked like a .22 caliber and there was no exit wound. I couldn't help but feel that it was a great loss to the community.

Atka

Sept 2, 2008 — Tuesday.

WHAT A REALLY GOOD TRIP OUT! We were only 45 minutes late out of Anchorage. PenAir assured me Vita was on board (3 times). In Dutch I went to collect my luggage to transfer to Atka on the Navajo. The cooler and box of books were there but no Vita, no gun, no big blue duffle with all my essentials! The baggage man said, "That's it, no more baggage." The agent at the desk was extremely anxious, as was I. She hurried off to see what happened. I told her "no dog, no passenger." She came back all smiles and said they had already loaded all three into the Navajo. I was the only passenger so the rest of the space was filled with freight. I squeezed by and sat where I could see all the instruments. Weather clear and sunny for a change, so easy in to Atka. I had forgotten how beautiful the soft green hills are.

Millie was there and I was happy to see her. I will get my currants and mushrooms to her today. I met the aide I'm replacing. She will go to Barrow. She told me who had been living in the quarters previously and that she had cleaned up as best she could. That sounded ominous. After Vita peed and peed we climbed into the old white van, the one with the flat tire the last visit. I noted there was one low tire this time as well.

I drove to this house I hated last time but assumed had improved. The holes in the walls and doors have been patched BUT the inner porch was full of sacked garbage. Rats had gotten in one bag, and the fish carcass I pulled free dropped 20 or 30 fat, centimeter-long maggots onto the floor. It stunk mightily and still does. Someone had cleaned fish on the counter and there were still pieces of fish anatomy on the board as well as slime and sand. More blood on the floor.

I could tell how much the aide must have done to make the interior livable. How she stood it here I do not know. At least the washer and dryer work. No clean sheets so I washed a set. When I pulled the bed from the wall to make it, I was appalled at the mess. I was so disgusted that I swept it up into many dustpans full and dumped it into the "play room." How can people live like that? I won't go on because it just makes me mad all over.

I have a shopping list that includes rubber gloves, dish soap, sponges with green mesh, and Chore Girls if the store has them. Also, when I got up this morning I found there was no heat. I am sure we are out of oil since that happened last time as well—some dispute about who pays—APIA or the village.

I tried to de-stench the garbage room. Clorox all around, and I moved the garbage outside. Of course, dogs got in it last night and now it is spread all over. At least it is outside. I really cannot live in filth. I will try to concentrate on what I do like out here. If it hadn't been for Vita I would have left on the next plane (two days from now).

Off to work if I can find what I did with the van keys.

9-3-08

WEDNESDAY—A QUIET day at the clinic—only 97 people live in Atka now. Millie came in for her job and we talked a lot. George Dirks, the former very good mayor, and his father both died, and then their house burned down in an electrical fire. I don't think this village will be the same without George.

I called Louis about the furnace problem. He is the wonderful skiff driver who took me through Amlia Pass one time—no easy feat. Arnold came and took the garbage—thank heaven. Rain poured through the mist all day and I began to feel at home. I took Vita for a one-hour run after work, and I do mean "run." She didn't stop once. We inspected the duck pond near the airport. No ducks. Must have been good smells, however; Vita's tail was a blur the entire time.

I came home to a warming house and had dinner of ham and Karen's sweet potato with pecans and a salad. Then I just sat and looked at the gorgeous green hills to the west. I think I etched them on my brain. I hope so. The curve is right where the creek has cut a deep ravine, and I know the creek is teeming with reds because I saw them jammed in the narrow part next to the beach on Nazan Bay.

9-6-08

SATURDAY—THINGS are very slow at the clinic. Janet saw only three patients in two weeks. I have seen two, with one scheduled for 1 p.m. after church today. One patient was a very cute 3-year-old whose dad had run a treble hook through his scalp while fishing for halibut (FROM THE BEACH! Where else could that be done?). It was superficial so I just cleaned it up and applied Steri-Strips.

Lots of activity to lengthen the landing strip. They are blasting rock out of the hill next to the pintail pot-hole—sadness—then crushing it and hauling it to the strip. Cheaper than barging it in. They work 24/7, and they must be careful, because I haven't seen any workers as patients. When they are done a 16-seater plane can land instead of the Navajo, which seats only six. Flights come on Monday, Wednesday and Friday plus any charter the outfit working on the runway gets in.

It has rained only one day this week. Clear and sunny again today. Vita and I went for a long walk in the hills the other side of the clinic yesterday. The creek is brimming with salmon. I ran Vita on a blind in one of the tarns. I thought the nice long swim would get rid of the stench of dried-on, rolled-in, dead salmon. The tarn is at least one foot more shallow than I remembered, and it was all running water with not a stroke of swim. Every one I came to was down about the same. The tundra crunched instead of the old pleasant squish I love. It was hard to find moss damp enough to yield berries. Took about an hour to gather a pint for Millie. (Irreplaceable Millie, without whom this village, and especially the clinic, could not function.) She has arthritis now, and every motion is painful to her.

I was pleased to find I did not get lost in the hills. The looked-for tarns were always right where I had left them a couple of years ago. Instead of the flocks of ptarmigan we flushed then, Vita nosed one lone bird out. They are usually all over town, but I haven't seen any here so far. I figured the foxes had been getting fat on them so didn't even take my gun on our walk.

I have been waiting for the boiler to heat up so I can take a shower. The electricity goes off at least once a day, and if I forget to push the re-set button, the boiler cools down. After our five-hour hike yesterday I was too tired to check it last night, because the water was hot enough to wash dishes.

Oh, I just remembered a delicious sight. As I was eating dinner and gazing out the window I saw a little girl dash across the tundra wearing a violent pink tutu! Like seeing a butterfly in the arctic! There must have been a special occasion. Certainly was for me.

Later: Only a three hour walk today. I saw a fellow at the clinic with hypertension and severe dermatitis of his hands, back, abdomen, arms and lower legs. Had my usual fight with the PickPoint, the newly installed medicine-dispensing horror machine. I finally cheated and opened the box by manual operation and got out what meds I had for him. Only 1% Hydrocort and he uses 3%. At least talked about other helpful things for dermatitis. Thence home and packed sandwiches and tried to get the 4-wheeler going. It started OK, though the choke lever is gone, but I couldn't remember how to get it into reverse so decided to be safe and drove the van over toward Korovin Bay on the Bering Sea side. Pulled off and walked the last ¼ mile because a good turn-around spot appeared. I walked down toward "Easter Egg Beach" with all the beautiful rocks, but the tide was in and I couldn't see them. There were so many salmon on the beach—another "gull buffet." Vita alternately rolled in them and chewed on them. She was so funny, running and playing in the surf like a

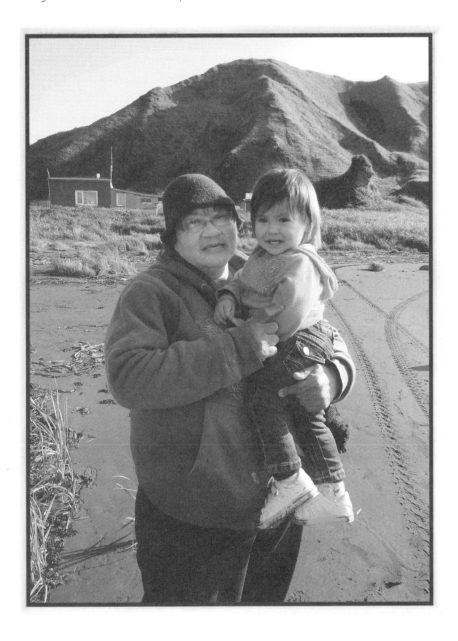

MILLIE PROKOPEUFF *and granddaughter* LIYANELLA PROKOPEUFF
at Korovin Beach, north of Atka village, July 2012.
Photo courtesy of Millie Prokopeuff.

little kid. I sat on a log to eat lunch and rest while she explored the beach grasses. On the way home I stopped at the edge of Korovin Lake so Vita could drink non-salty water and saw fresh reindeer tracks—lots of them. Saw 4-wheeler tracks, too, so the entire town knows by now. Didn't see any animals.

Too tired to write so will fix dinner and go to bed. Glad I got the washing dried in time to make the bed.

9-9-08

TUESDAY—BACK TO NORMAL Atka weather, with rain and gusting northwest winds. The house shook a little last night but less this morning. I tried to walk along the beach to be in the lee under the bank, but it blew sand so hard I felt I was in a sanding box. Vita had her usual swell time.

Work was busy although everything takes so long—can't find things I need, new fax number for the PickPoint that no one bothered to tell me. I will try to look at it as a lesson in patience. People are actually starting to come in to the clinic to be seen, and that pleases me. Making referrals and transportation arrangements is a nightmare. Stupid federal agency says "Weather" is not an excuse for non-travel on appointment days. I try to explain that we are over 1,300 miles from the appointment place and it is over water. If the plane does not fly are we to swim, walk on water? I hate bureaucracy and its disapproval of thinking.

The dental crew that was supposed to arrive yesterday is stranded in Dutch—the plane couldn't get out to bring them here. I hope PenAir tries again today. I am sure it will jam the little clinic up, and the phone will ring nonstop when the village gets the word. Actually, the village will hear the plane if it gets in, and all will know the dentists are on board.

Millie and I plus two of her children moved all the heavy dental supplies from the Bingo hall over to the clinic last week. We had to clear one exam room out and store things in the shower and an adjacent shed. We couldn't have done it without the family help. Millie's arthritis was much worse the next day. I wonder what it will be like to have the x-ray machine set up in the waiting room. Perhaps I will receive a lesson in welcoming chaos.

9-10-08

WEDNESDAY—THE DENTAL CREW still hasn't made it out of Dutch. The weather here is fine—no wind or rain this morning. Millie showed me how to use the Internet to actually see the weather in Dutch via weather-cam. FOG—couldn't see from one end of the runway to the other. The dentist and the dental techs now plan to work over the weekend if they get in before then.

The electricity just went off. Glad I had already made tea. When I pulled the sheet off the window hoping for more light to find the flashlight, I could see rain and fog appearing, so I bet the dentists don't make it today either. The phone is out as well so no point in going to the clinic in the dark. Worst of all, now I have no music! The tape player is battery powered but the speakers are not. And the jigsaw puzzle is impossible by flashlight. The only lights I see are from a fishing boat and one from the quarry. At least I hear a 4-wheeler, so someone is on the way to the power plant.

. .

Later, at work: Power back on. I spent an hour on the phone trying to fix Titiana Zaochney's travel plans—her third try to get to town for consults. Her appointment is for Monday in Anchorage. PenAir flies on Friday and Saturday. Knowing the weather, Titiana is aware that she cannot count on getting out just because she has a reservation. She is trying to get a reservation for Friday because if that flight doesn't get out, she has a second chance on Saturday. Medicaid does not pay full price for tickets and will not pay for tickets booked by a patient. I suppose that prevents patients from flying first class. The airline does not want to issue a ticket to Medicaid if it can sell that seat to a person for the full price. For some reason, when Medicaid calls PenAir to book Titiana's Friday travel, all the seats have been sold. When Titiana calls for herself, PenAir has plenty of seats available Of course, if she books a seat, Medicaid won't pay and she is stuck with the price of the ticket. I think my blood pressure is rising.

Millie is still home mornings waiting for her joints to loosen up, so I am learning the coffee drill. (1) Run the water at least 15 minutes before loading the coffee machine. The pipes in this old building are lead. The lead-laden water has to bleed out to get fresh. (2) Only one scoop of coffee. (3) Don't forget to turn the upper unit on to heat water for tea. I miss her company and expertise.

Sally Swetzof came in to retrieve the sunglasses she left here yesterday. She is feeling much better and we're both happy for that. She introduced me to her daughter, Crystal, who teaches a bilingual class in Aleut/English at the school. Sally's pride is apparent.

And now I can see Cake Island in the bay. I looked at the weather cam of Dutch and it looks pretty good. Maybe the dentists will get in tomorrow.

. .

NOON: NOW I CAN'T even see Cake.

9-11-08

THURSDAY—THICK fog this morning but the sun is burning it off very rapidly. I looked at Dutch weather cam and it looks iffy. The dentists have canceled and now I understand why no one called to make an appointment. No one bothers until the dentists get in. Smart. But now we will have to lug all that heavy equipment back into storage. While I was out in the hills with Vita after work yesterday I heard a plane make a pass at the strip. I couldn't see it through the fog, which was right down to the deck, and I was less than half a mile away. It must have been a charter because PenAir has more sense. At my quarters less than 100 yards from the beach of Nazan Bay, I could not see the beach or the bay.

I find I like the effect of fog. It is like the squelch on the plane radios, cutting off extraneous noises and distractions, allowing for all-important centering. I am reminded of Elizabeth Bishop, whose writing room in Brazil had no windows so that she could avoid distraction. Jung is so right about the importance of individuation, which I think must come gradually, building a firm foundation before it is able to make even the smallest leap. So we stutter on through the fog hoping the deviation on our personal compass is correct. Oh, here comes a poem into my head—

ALEUT ELDER

Thick fog surrounds me.
I am a mist bound fetus,
always becoming.

And now to study my continuing medical education course on the clinical management of atrial fibrillation.

9-12-08

FRIDAY—THAT PLANE I heard in the fog on the 10th was a charter, and it was taking off after having landed. Although I was only a quarter of a mile from the airport, I couldn't see it through the fog. The plane made it, but I'm glad I wasn't aboard. They sure didn't have the 200-feet-above-ground-level and two miles required, and there certainly isn't any instrument landing system out here.

The dentists who canceled have decided to try again next week, and we have decided to leave all their boxes and trunks here instead of moving them out and then back in again, considering they might not make it then either.

On the home front, the 55-gallon gasoline drum with a hand pump on it next to my porch is completely empty. Instead of paying the pump price at Atka Fishing Association, I hand-pump it into a five-gallon can from the barrel and then pour the gas into the van tank, thus saving much money. Authorization to fill the drum must come from APIA in

Anchorage, after which dear man of many talents Arnold will pick up the empty drum, cart it off and fill it at the main tank, and bring it back here. Arnold only works that job 8–12 since he has another job in the afternoon. This means Anchorage has to arrange this with him before noon. Naturally the person to authorize it is "unavailable" and who knows when she will retrieve this message. Millie and I started working on this two days ago and are now looking at the weekend. But wait!—Anchorage just called and gave me the authorization number! One for the home team!

9-13-08

SATURDAY—CLEAR—I can see stars for the first time. This will be Titiana's third try to go to ANMC (Alaska Native Medical Center) in Anchorage. Hope she makes it. I slept in until 6:30. I was going to make mossberry pancakes for breakfast but will save that for tomorrow when I will splurge and have coffee instead of tea for breakfast. I am definitely in the going-home phase—especially with this weekend to enjoy. I don't have to deal with federal agencies for 48 hours! I brought the little electronic scale home to weigh my luggage for the PenAir manifest. I even remembered to categorize into essential (me, Vita, gun) and non-essential (cooler, books, CD's, tapes, clothes). With load limits, luggage frequently gets left here.

After work last night I decided to try to find the track to the old village site. I had thought the original village was on Old Harbor where the clinic is, but it was on the Bering Sea side of the island somewhere. Nazan Bay, where the village is now, is on the Pacific side. I love being able to walk from the Pacific to the Bering Sea. Yesterday I must have taken the wrong trail. It petered out in a bog. I skirted that and climbed upslope where a rainbow appeared with one end anchored in Korovin Lake and the other right on the village with the strip and Nazan Bay under the arc. Well worth the climb.

I had secreted a couple of bumpers into my pack along with the essential radio so did a blind and a mark for Vita, to her great joy. She does love the tundra, and I love to see her excellence in being who she is. We trekked happily downslope in wind and rain, headed for home and dinner.

This is Saturday, so I will pack a lunch and hike over to the Bering Sea side and beach-comb to the southwest for a change. I hope I can find the bridge over the creek. It is too deep to ford, plus there are so many salmon in it that they would probably knock me over. I do love to see them, though. It used to make me sad, all coming home to die. But now they have shown that the fry (their children) are sustained by all those dead bodies, grow, and get strong to repeat the cycle.

9-14-08

Sunday—Vita was such a pill in the morning that I took her along to the clinic while I checked e-mail and Dutch weather (expect no plane again today), then hiked up the old hydro-plant trail just to let her run. It has been kind of a nothing day. I have begun to cherish them because I finally know they are necessary for things to "grow." PenAir did cancel, and Titiana didn't get out again. As I went for my afternoon walk I saw a twin charter (Ace) get in.

I have now had two good nights' sleep in succession— what a difference that makes! I have done my personal wash in preparation for tomorrow's departure and made real Gevalia's coffee plus have the mossberries for pancakes, and I

even have two eggs left. I shall have a feast! If I continue to
feel good I will take the Korovin trip I planned yesterday. Will
see if I brave the 4-wheeler for transport.

. .

Dɪᴅ ɪᴛ! Wᴇ ʜᴀᴅ ᴀ ᴠᴇʀʏ ɴɪᴄᴇ ᴅᴀʏ. The 4-wheeler had a flat
tire, but some nice gentleman led me to the place at the Atka
Fisherman's Association where air was available. Getting it
there was much faster than dragging over the hill to that other
place near the garage on the hill. It must be a slow leak,
because the tire is still tight after our trip.

Vita ran all the way out to Korovin and back. Easy trip as
far as getting past the lake, until I got to the creek. I was
afraid I would get stuck in the creek trying to cross over it to
the left at Korovin Bay so took the road across the bridge.
Mistake! I checked the planks out before trying to cross, then
made it, but at the last turn in the path buried the right front
tire in a large hole and I was so stuck. I tried to lever it out
with a piece of lumber I found. No dice. Put it in 4-wheel-
drive. No dice. Only two wheels on the ground and I couldn't
push it even in neutral. I sat at the cross-path and ate lunch
trying to keep Vita away. She had found a wonderful pile of
decomposed salmon to roll in and was entirely covered on
both sides. Phew! After about an hour a man drove up on a
dirt bike and offered to help. He sat on the 4-wheeler and
leaned over the uphill side in reverse while I pushed from the
front. Out it came. I was very happy not to have to call Millie
on the radio and have the entire village know I was stuck. It
turns out my helper is from Homer, at the end of the Kenai
Peninsula south of Anchorage, and knows Findlay and the

rest of the Abbotts, dear friends from Yukon Island out in Kachemak Bay. We had old home week. He is working construction on the new AFA place near the little dock.

After I got the beast turned around and back on the main path I parked it and Vita and I set off for Martin Cove. Great walk on a very nice day. Saw two big flocks of ducks. I bet they taste fishy. Lots of fox tracks. Sat on a rock and just enjoyed the view while eating a Snickers bar, then hiked back to the 4-wheeler and set off for home. Put Vita in the lake on the way and tried to wash the rotten fish out. She ate a big dinner at home and collapsed. I went over to the office to try to check e-mail. Of course the Internet was down. Hope it is up by morning. I will pack tonight and be ready in case the flight gets in.

9-17-08

WEDNESDAY—MADE IT home but not without the usual drama. I got up early to wash the linens—there is only one set of sheets. I hung it all to dry in the furnace room. Really cleaned the stinky mud room/inner porch and finally got rid of the stench there. Organized my luggage and managed to fit the Extratuf box into my blue duffle so there was only the duffle, gun-case, cooler and dog crate. Had extra food in case I was weathered in, so wrapped it in newspaper and put it in the cooler at the last minute. I got to work on time and the Internet was actually on. I got the weather cam from Dutch and the weather was clear! Tied up loose ends at the office and left a note for the next person. PenAir called to tell me they were on schedule for 1:30. I had weighed all my gear, so gave PenAir the figures plus my weight, then dashed home for lunch before we left. Hah! No plane, no plane. I had the VHF radio on and finally heard the pilot call on approach about 3:30. We are one time zone west of Dutch, which meant it was 4:30 there. It is a two-hour flight from Atka to Dutch, and my connecting flight was to leave for Anchorage at 5:30. We got off a little after 4 Atka time. I managed to give the clinic keys to Annette, my replacement, and even remembered to give her the van keys. After we were under way I discovered I still had the radio in my pack. Oh well, two more are at quarters and I'll mail it. Nice pilot let Vita sit next to me instead of in her crate. It was an easy flight at 9,500 feet. Pilot put it on autopilot and read a book.

I had hoped the airline would hold the 5:30 flight for us but the Saab was not there when we arrived. Figured I was stuck overnight and who could know what the weather would be tomorrow. Went to the counter and explained I'd missed my flight, at which point the agent treated me as though I had overslept or stayed too long in the bar. Dutch had been socked in for five days, and PenAir had an extra section coming but it had only 30 seats and there were at least 45 people trying to get out. I set her straight that PenAir was two hours late getting to Atka, which was the reason I had missed my flight.

About that time I saw Clare Lattimore, the FNP (family nurse practitioner) from Dutch, sitting next to her dog crate waiting to get out. That relieved my stress. She said I could stay at her place if we didn't get out. Good to see her. Her dog, Rosie, is a Nova Scotia Tolling Dog and a good friend of Vita's. (I once had the opportunity to train with a man who had a tolling dog. We were out by the beach on Unalaska Lake practicing blinds and marks with not a bird in sight. He asked if I would like to see his dog "in action." Of course I said yes, so we hunkered down in the bushes and he sent his dog to the beach where she put on her act. She ran up and down the beach excitedly and leapt about like a ballerina. Suddenly birds began to come from all over to see what all the excitement was about. It was an amazing demonstration that I have never forgotten.)

Now, back in the waiting room, I was starving, but neither Clare nor I wanted to go into the bar to eat. It is smoke-filled and very noisy with sports TV and a lot of drunks. She shared her cashews and I shared my remaining home-baked "vanishing oatmeal cookies." And then, oh joy, they called her name to be one of the 30. I held my breath and then they called my name! I checked in, took Vita out to pee, and we were off. I got home with all my luggage and Vita, which is practically unheard of.

So good to be home.

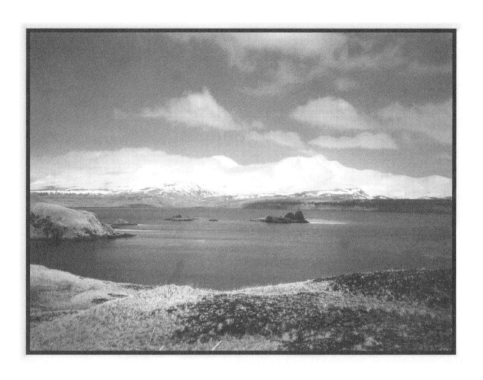

FROM THE HILL *above the "old village" of Atka,*
looking across Nazan Bay toward Korovin volcano.

St. George

Dec. 27, 2008 — Saturday.

"BONE" LEKANOF DROVE ME INTO TOWN yesterday from the airport. He is the great beachcomber who was raised here on the island. He waxed eloquent on the way to town. I liked the story of the orca tooth best, but he also found a huge walrus tusk one time.

It was a typical travel day. First PenAir canceled Cold Bay and Sand Point, then they moved our departure from noon to 1:30 p.m. Finally, they announced that the plane was going to St. Paul but the weather was too bad to go to St. George. If we wanted to fly all that way out there just to return home they would try, but it didn't look good. I would have gone home in a minute, but I can't do that when I replace someone. I remember a time in Nikolski when I was three days late getting out. I rejoiced at the sight of the plane but then was dismayed to learn that my replacement had decided it wasn't worth the chance of not getting in and I had to stay much longer. So off I went. We got in to St. Paul and waited to see if the pilot would try St. George. Hooray—except that dear PenAir didn't bring any luggage. So here I am with no toothbrush or clean clothes, etc. The airline promises tomorrow, but I know how that goes.

The aide I am replacing left a pot of very good turkey soup, and I found a candy bar. The store is closed Sunday so tomorrow I will root around for food. I am glad I hand-carried the laptop and my early Dutch material—journals and letters and whatnot.

I have already seen one patient with a supraorbital contusion. All nervous systems checked out OK.

Tuesday

I DID SUCCESSFUL blood draws this morning, but the villagers know the weather and if it isn't flyable they won't come in —they know the plane won't get in and they will just have to come in again and be stuck once more. PenAir got as far as St. Paul with my luggage but the crosswind was too strong here for the plane to try it. I'm getting tired of turkey soup. I went to the store yesterday and bought what I thought was chicken and noodles. Turned out it was only chicken "flavored" noodles.

I saw only a couple of patients yesterday. The one with chronic obstructive pulmonary disease (COPD) I saw on Sunday with low-grade fever is doing better on Azithromycin. He is still smoking a pack of cigarettes a day, however.

Most of the work is getting the clinic in shape. Seven itinerants have been here in the past few months. Therefore there is no continuity of care, which is invaluable. New office manager —Grace— is both smart and well-organized so will make a huge difference. I think I was on my own the last time I was here. It is sort of like Nikolski, where I do everything from cleaning the clinic to making appointments and travel arrangements plus all the medical practice that needs attention.

Jan. 5, 2009

MONDAY—WHAT APPROPRIATE TAPES I'm listening to this morning: Dohnanyi—trio, op 10, quintet, op 26, no. 7, and Piano Quintet in E-flat minor. It fits the unrest I'm feeling. When I took a walk yesterday in gale-force winds I couldn't help stopping all the time to drink in the sight of the tempestuous seas offshore. It was like looking at what was going on inside of me except that it was beautiful.

The water was slate gray with brilliant whitecaps and yards of white froth near the cliffs. Then the sun came out and changed the color of the water to a greenish cast that gave it all greater depth. I guess I am in a period of transition, because I'm thinking of retiring from this work I love. Of course I don't like all the uncertainties. I always find it hard to wait things out. Find I'm returning to that quote that I never get quite right about how the point at the very outer limit of faith and the one at the start of despair are identical. Time for work.

Nikolski Hills

This time of year the sly hills wear brown,
light, dark, tan, mottled, sandy—
like a huge awakening grizzly,
sun glinting off silver guard hairs.

Under the tawny insulating mat
secret summer blossoms spread
their roots in readiness
for the Fourth of July when
with one great shake of the giant pelt,
they will explode in every color
on a new green carpet.

Whole fields of lupine await
their entrance cue
to burst forth in
acres of blue and green where
we roll down and over
in Pentecostal fervor.

Nikolski—on the way

July 16, 2009 — Thursday.

WHILE I SAT IN THE DEPARTURE LOUNGE in Anchorage reading the morning paper and doing the puzzles—and listening to flights being delayed—quite a few people came to say hello to Vita. The nice counter person had said I could keep her with me and they would come to get her with her crate when the plane was ready. One kid kept taking her on the leash around the room. Another passenger told me Vita was a "therapy dog," calming all the anxious passengers. The man next to me wanted to pet her and showed me pictures of his dog.

At 11:30, two hours after our scheduled departure, they came with her crate and we finally left. Two hours to King Salmon for refueling and another two hours on to Dutch—good weather, no turbulence! When I deplaned at the airport I saw signs all over directing smokers outside and no closer to the doors than 20 feet. The place still stinks of stale cigarette smoke but at least I can see across the hall, which is a big improvement.

Abi was here to greet me and I dashed out to see if the Goose had already left for Nikolski. It had been due to leave at 1:30 and it was now 4 p.m.. Alas, fog in Nikolski, so the flight was canceled. Dear Abi helped me load all my gear into her truck and we set off for the Grand Aleutian. Word was that the hotel no longer accepts dogs, but we have been here before and the manager said OK. I had dinner with Abi at her place and cooked my freezer-burned salmon to add to Vita's food. Eagles were everywhere, all fighting for fish. Vita loves the tundra and went running on her own, inhaling all the good smells.

After dinner I checked into the hotel, moved all the gear in and took two boxes to the cooler overnight. PenAir says it will try 1:30 tomorrow, and I will check in around noon.

Too tired for more—out the window I see fish jumping in Margaret Bay. People fishing, but I don't see anyone catching except one sea lion that seems to be doing rather well.

7-17-09

FRIDAY—AFTER A wonderful full night's sleep I took Vita out for a walk and got within 10 feet of two gorgeous eagles sitting on poles overlooking the bay. Didn't have my camera.

I went to Amelia's Restaurant for breakfast, and the cook recognized me and came right over to the table. She said she was happy to see me back as they could always use really good doctors in town. I told her I was just stuck trying to get in to Nikolski. How nice to be greeted so enthusiastically after all these years.

The plane isn't leaving until 1:30 this afternoon—if it leaves then—so I have decided to go to the clinic and have the sutures from my right carpal tunnel surgery removed. I know I can't do it alone with my left hand. I will be nine days post-op instead of 10 but should be OK. If they are swamped, I will stay and work until noon.

7-19-09

Sunday—still in Dutch—Yesterday was a disaster. My hand kept me awake all night after I hiked up a very steep hill where I had to use both hands to keep from rolling down. Then when I called to check on my flight they said it was only 200 feet below minimums and they were going to try for 1 p.m. It was then 11:30 so I threw my bags together, got the boxes from the hotel cooler (fresh veggies and strawberries for Scott and Agrafina) and with kennel and dog took the five-minute shuttle to the airport. I checked kennel, blue duffle, and my old cardboard planer box full of dog food and whatever else I could stuff in. It's covered with duct tape from all its trips, but the rope handle is still intact. I also checked the cooler plus the heavy backpack with my laptop, Sudoku book, and emergency breakfast bars. Waited, waited, waited. The pilot finally came out and said it was really thick fog almost to the water but he would recheck and not cancel until 4 or so.

I decided to take Vita for a walk and look for more of the abundant tundra flowers. Found some new ones up on Standard Oil Hill. Abi had identified three different kinds of "spike" orchids I found earlier—a fuchsia-colored one called the "Purple" or "Showy" orchid (*Dactylorhiza aristata*), a tall, very fragrant one, the "White Bog" or "Bog Candles" orchid (*Plantanthera dilatata*), and a green bog orchid known locally as "Cornflower" (*Plantanthera convallariaefolia*). I feel so smart.

When I got back, it was almost 4 and the flight was canceled, so I returned to the hotel and checked in again. I was too tired to go to Abi's for dinner—her friend Steve is there to keep her company anyway. Had dinner here (very good crab cakes), checked my e-mail and crashed into bed by 8:45. I slept until 7.

Peat is living at the Senior Center here so I will try to get over to see him before I leave. Better get at it. It is already 10 a.m.

. .

I HAVE TO WRITE ABOUT THIS EXCITEMENT. Through my window I could see a man catch a nice red salmon. He killed it and left it on the beach while he went farther along to try a new spot. Later I saw him running so got up to see why. An eagle was eating his fish as fast as it could. He threw a rock but it landed short and the eagle tried to take off with the whole fish in its talons. The eagle didn't get a good grip and dropped the salmon into the bay, but near shore. The man managed to snag it and then just picked up and went home. Oh, much better than television!

7-20-09

*M*ONDAY—THIS is the Dutch I remember—pelting rain, strong winds, clouds almost down to the deck. Obviously, Nikolski canceled again. Abi took me to the library where I got e-mail and books. Saw Peat in the Senior Center, which is right next to the library. Cora works at the library, so saw her as well. Both seem fine. Got the right spelling for fried bread. It is time for tea while I rejoice in the fact that I am not here in a tent.

7-21-09

*T*UESDAY—ANOTHER fine day in Dutch. Wind gusts blowing "cat's paws" across the bay while homeward-bound reds leap out of the waves trying to shed their sea lice. Not many eagles lurking this morning. I'm glad I got a good book from the library yesterday. I will have to patch my rain pants if I go out today. My knees got wet while airing Vita. I already bought a roll of duct tape.

7-22-09

WEDNESDAY—THIS marks a week of waiting. "No Fog" must be like "Godot." Abi finally managed to get out for Anchorage at 7 last night. I am scheduled for 1 p.m. When I called PenAir at 10:45 this morning the woman was pretty sure we wouldn't get to Nikolski today, so I called the clinic to see if I could use the car. The PA who took my sutures out had the little car and was happy to let me use it until closing time at 4 p.m. Whoopee! I drove to the library and checked e-mail and let everyone know I was still in Dutch—needed a full hour to get everything cleared up. Drove home, had a bowl of soup, and then took Vita out toward Pyramid Peak up behind Captain's Bay. It was wonderful! Great marks and blinds all over the place. Even did a double blind. One to the top of a hill, followed by one at the bottom. She nailed both!

The fog here suddenly lifted and I worried about possibly missing a Nikolski flight. It was 3:30 p.m. by this time, so I drove to the airport and saw the canceled sign. I dashed back to Iliuliuk Lake, near the high school, and parked in the Methodist church parking lot next to the lake, just past two float plane tie-downs. Where else could you see two float plane tie-downs in a church parking lot? From the point farther out I saw a super blind from the other side. It would take Vita into the lake, through a swampy weedy area, back into the lake, over an eagle-inhabited island, back into the lake, over a grassy hook and finally back into the lake for the "bird" on the near shore. She popped (unsolicited look back for direction) once and I got a correction, but the rest was great.

7-27-09

MONDAY—NIKOLSKI at last—I finally made it out of Dutch last Thursday in the Goose, which I love. The flight was held for "February," a 300-pound Samoan (the one who sent for a whole pig and had a Samoan pig feast for the village a couple of years ago). The plane was loaded but he didn't show. Did they then add 300 pounds of cargo? Of course not. There were only four of us and Vita. I even told them I would leave the kennel there to save pounds, since she travels just fine without it. Anyhow, after being shut out for over a week, we landed and found that PenAir did not even bring the mail or any cargo or luggage. What an outfit! Meds for patients were in the mail. This time I was smart enough, or finally experienced enough, to have packed six days of dog food in my carry-on plus a toothbrush and change of underwear and sox. I had also put the bottle brush and cough drops for Agrafina there. I hand-carried the cooler as well. The Grand Aleutian had stored it in the freezer instead of the cooler, thus freezing the fresh strawberries, lettuce, tomatoes, and bok choy. (Agrafina made strawberry smoothies so all was not lost.) Vita's cooked freezer-burned salmon was OK, so I may be able to stretch her food if no plane gets in in the next few days. PenAir promised us a second flight on Thursday but I didn't believe it. We had clear skies here on Friday—no plane.

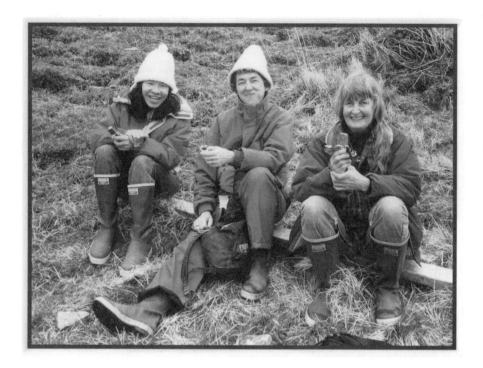

From left, AGRAFINA, NANCY *and* MARLAINE, *on a visit
to the cattle ranch at Chernofski.*

Sunday, no plane. And of course today when there is a scheduled flight the fog is down to the deck.

My arrangements had been made in Anchorage this time, and I was booked at the lodge. Sean, the charter operator at the lodge, came over and introduced himself and offered me a ride. I had the new clinic van, however (can't believe the grandeur), so I just drove out after giving the cooler to Scott and telling him of the freezer disaster. Scott has two new Chessies, Whirlwind's grandson "Breaker" (I'm sure that has a very different meaning for him than for me—it is such a bad trait in field trials), and a 4-month-old pup named "Sasha."

7-28-09

TUESDAY—GORGEOUS day today—no fog or wind—but I checked on the weather channel and Dutch is socked in tight, so no freight again today. I have started bringing Vita to work with me in the afternoons. She waits in the van until 4, when we go out and do walking singles. I have quit blinds since she has started to pop and I don't have her collar or the transmitter to correct her. I saw one patient this morning for drug refills. Agrafina and I installed new batteries in the smoke alarms so all four are now functioning. I found one new alarm in the cupboard, and Sean came over from the lodge to install it in the furnace room. I checked all the emergency lights and they are OK.

7-29-09

WEDNESDAY—THE drive to work this morning was wonderful. As I headed out of the yard I saw a group of wild horses about 50 yards from the inn, three mares with various size foals all tame and unconcerned as I passed. Then in the next 50 feet were the fox vixen with her four kits, in the rubble of the barn that blew down when someone forgot to close the doors. I do love to see foxes and hear their croak of a bark. Down the hill, where the creek runs into the bay, seagulls and eagles were scouting for fish. (The red run is on, and Scott used a small seine net and got more than 200 for the village.) Then up the hill, past the refurbished Russian Orthodox church gleaming white, with fresh new blue paint on the domes. I was skeptical at first when I heard that Barbara Sweetland Smith had gotten a grant to renew "war-damaged churches in the Aleutians." I knew the Japanese had not damaged the Nikolski church, nor the ones in St. Paul, Atka, or St. George. They had bombed Dutch Harbor, so I thought the damage to the Unalaska church was from the bombing. Then I learned that it was our troops who shot at the crosses and broke in and ruined the interiors, while the villagers were trying to survive in Southeast Alaska after their forced, hasty evacuation. Indeed it was war damage. War teaches destruction. The church in Atka—including all the birth, death and other records—was ordered burned by our military, to prevent the invading Japanese from using it. Really!

I drove past the church and on to the clinic through a maze of hopping rabbits that apparently live under the Conexes. I am sure the foxes never grow hungry.

7-29-09

WEDNESDAY—SO FAR I have seen only one patient per day here, but then the total population is only about two dozen. I am trying to do all the end-of-the-month paperwork to send to Anchorage. Thank goodness the clinic has no vaccine, because the little drug refrigerator has a freezer with a temperature of about 28–30 degrees. I think we could keep it in the food refrigerator in the kitchen. No babies in town anyway.

I keep seeing beautiful blinds for Vita, both water and land, but am afraid to run them without her collar, which is in my undelivered luggage. There is one gorgeous water blind —a shoreline with three points and lots of distance. I do mostly walking singles because I have only one bumper with me; the rest are with the collar and transmitter. She gets very excited even about singles.

I saw a group of old squaw ducks in the bay. It has been so long since I've seen them that I had to look them up in the bird book to be sure. I pick new bog orchids every day when I take Vita out. I remember those fragrant "Ladies Tresses" so well from the 10-day cruise we took with Marlaine on the *Spirit*. I put them in my pillowcase every night.

7-31-09

FRIDAY—THIS morning I got up early and checked the weather. Clear in all quadrants, and clear in Dutch as well. Gulped tea and started packing. After breakfast I looked and we were socked in again. I am happily in the clinic listening to Mendelssohn, which Agrafina showed me how to do on the computer. One of the fox kits keeps traipsing along outside the windows, and all the rabbits are under cover. There is a one-hour time difference between here and Anchorage so the Open in the retriever trials is already well under way. Vita was to be the last dog to run, but I don't have to worry about that anymore.

The lodge people are going halibut fishing today. Dear Sean cuts the line on any fish over four feet long. I like him. The big ones are all breeding females. The males never get over 50–75 pounds.

What's this? A patient? No, it is Agrafina and Scott. We had a good visit and after they left, Agrafina called to tell me that PenAir was sending a plane! They were loading at the time. I locked everything up and tore back to the lodge. Cindy, the charter operator's wife, had made good thick homemade soup but I could only smell it while I got things ready. I let Vita out and crammed the last of my things into the box and duffle. I filled the little cooler with halibut that Sean had told me I could have. I threw everything in the back of the van, slurped the soup, and took Cindy along as we tore for the airport. We were to pick up the communication man on the way. The plane landed as we picked him up so there was no wait. I had time to talk to Grace, the CHA I replaced—told her I had no warning so things were not as shipshape as I would have liked, and went over the important things. They finished loading the plane and Vita flew up the ladder. Everyone was impressed. The bottom of the door is about 6½ feet above ground. There were only three of us headed for Dutch, so there was plenty of room for luggage. I was so happy to realize I would get there in time to catch one of the two late-afternoon flights to Anchorage.

It was a beautiful flight along the back side of Umnak. There was a stiff crosswind on arrival, but the pilot landed on one wheel and kept it nice and straight. But alas—no seats on either of the flights going out.

I met Abi coming in on one of the flights. Her luggage was to be on the next one, so we visited until it came in. As we were about to leave, the very nice counter woman came over to tell me there was no standby space but she had confirmed me on the 1 p.m. flight tomorrow. Abi drove me to the hotel where they had a room, thank goodness. I said goodbye to Abi, fed Vita, and dropped in to the "Cheerful" for a margarita. It was after 6 p.m. by then. I took Vita for a walk and felt tired so just had yogurt and a cereal bar for dinner. Now I am ready for bed after listening to Bill Moyer's discussion of national health care. He was excellent. Tonight's music is Mozart: Piano Concerto in B flat, plus one in C and one in D. (I shocked everyone in Nikolski with my CD of Leon Redbone.)

8-1-09

SATURDAY—WHAT is better than lying in bed looking at fog out the window while listening to Jaqueline du Pre playing Schumann's Cello Concerto in A minor—just right, and I understand why Bo cried when he heard she had multiple sclerosis. PenAir line is busy, busy, busy. If I don't get out, I will trek to the library and check e-mail. Ah, Schumann! I am reading *The Other,* by David Guterson, and both the music and the fog seem to fit that. In other words, my mood—tranquil longing.

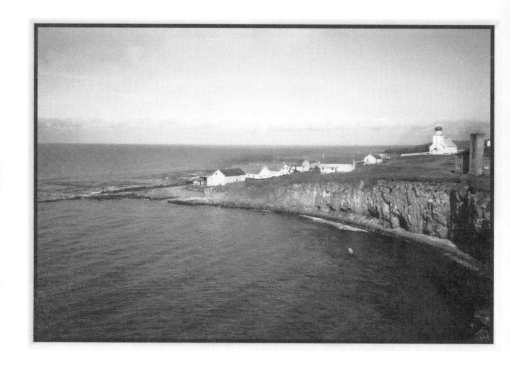

ST. GEORGE VILLAGE, *2002.*

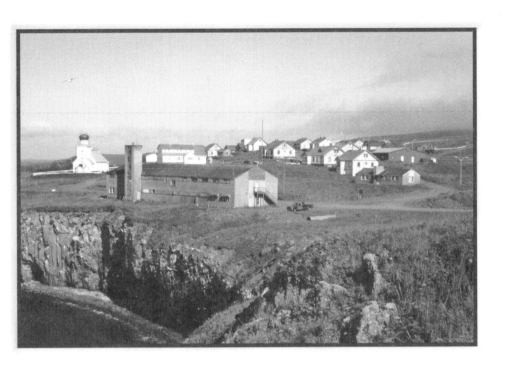

St George (on the way)

Oct. 4, 2009 — Sunday.

I WAS TO HAVE GONE TO ST. GEORGE last Thursday, September 24. I spent several hours waiting in the departure lounge reading until they canceled the flight due to "mechanical." Took a cab back home and returned on Friday to try again. This time I managed to get out, stopped in King Salmon for gas and to wait out the fog in St. Paul, and finally took off. I don't know how the pilot got there through the murk. We broke out at less than 200 feet over the water. He corrected to line up with the runway a scant 200 yards away and made it in. Next step, St. George? I checked the weather, waited, checked the weather, waited, checked the weather, until the pilot decided the plane couldn't get in to St. George and would return to Anchorage. I was going to stay. It had taken four hours to get to St. Paul and if I went home I would have to do it again on Saturday. Then the pilot said that sometimes they could get in to St. George and not St. Paul. This would then leave me stuck in St. Paul, so I went back to the plane and back to Anchorage.

Did things all over again Friday but the weather looked better. The plane easily got in to St. Paul this time, but held there for St. George for two hours and then canceled. This time I decided to stick it out in St. Paul. I called Jessica, the manager of the clinic there, and asked if I could stay. She welcomed me—said they could always use me, and I could stay in quarters. When she came out to pick me up, Pauline Rukovishnikof was along. I was so glad to see her, especially because her husband had recently died. I had wonderful turkey soup for dinner with her and her family. I invited Pauline for dinner the following night so she could taste my caribou meat loaf. I felt happy to be able to reciprocate.

There are no scheduled flights to St. George until next Thursday, unless they feel guilty about not getting anyone there for a week and add an extra flight earlier. I was scheduled to see patients here on Monday but was free until then. I had a walk out to the reef rookery and sadly noted the lack of foxes—found out later that the city had installed fox-proof garbage cans so all the foxes moved out to the tundra. I miss them.

Just as I was getting ready to see patients on Monday, PenAir called to say that if I wanted to go to St. George, I had better bring my luggage NOW. I dropped everything, threw things back in the bags and got a ride to the airport in time. I met the pilot, Bob Reeve Jr., one of the Reeve Aleutian Airways Reeves. He had gone to school with my son Ben and asked how he was. It does something to an old Aleutian traveler to know there is a Reeve in the cockpit. I just knew we would get in, and we did.

Grace Merculief, the new clinic manager, met me and drove me to the Aikow Inn because the health aide was in the quarters at the clinic. Aiko is Aleut for fox so I knew I would be right at home. Both silver and white foxes roam the streets all hours. In season the hotel is crammed with birders from all over the world, but the birding season is over so it was nearly empty and I had my choice of rooms. I took a corner room with a view of the city dock, where I could see baby seals learning to swim.

The Aikow has a library just inside the front door—three walls covered with books, many leather-bound in locked cases. *We*, by Lindberg, *Moment in Peking*, Newcomb's *Popular Astronomy*, *Tess of the d'Urbervilles*, and many more. What was a library of this kind doing in the middle of the Bering Sea? The mystery is right up there with the photograph of a string quartet in St. Paul that I ran across in the university museum in Fairbanks. (I found out that the first two floors of the inn were built in the 1930s by the Fouke Company for personnel involved in the fur seal harvest. The third floor was added much later.)

This library has leather chairs and davenport, reminding me of old pictures I have seen of men's clubs. On the walls above the bookcases are interesting pictures of St. George in the past as well as maps and pictures of flowers found on the island. In front of a window is a large table with a partially completed complex jigsaw puzzle full of musical instruments. There is a rug on the floor and several smaller bookshelves full of well-read paperbacks. It is a most comfortable room.

Continuing to explore I found a marvelous kitchen on the first floor with room for several parties to cook. Utile because there is no restaurant in the village. There were two huge refrigerators, two stoves, plus microwave ovens and cupboards galore with room for utensils and pots and pans. There is a small dining area, too, as well as a laundry room down the hall. All nicely planned—and the big plus is that it is always warm down there.

When I was choosing my room I noticed that every room had a small corner shelf that held a paper icon, holy water and a candle. I asked Marge Lestenkof, the caretaker, about that. She said they kept having complaints from guests about raucous parties in the night, with loud banging and crashing. None of the guests admitted guilt, and after the complaints persisted with many changes of guests they decided they had a poltergeist in the building. Marge installed the shelves in every room and they have had no problems since. I liked the inn even better after hearing this story.

Last night a marine biologist moved in next door. I will now clothe myself a little better on my trips to the bathroom down the hall. He is putting tracking devices on female seals. He says the mother seals used to be able to leave their pups for a few hours to feed themselves and could then return to nurse them, but now, because we have taken all the pollock on which the mothers feed, it may take them more than a week to find food. By the time they return, many of the pups have died. Interesting conversation on the decline of seals, putrefaction of the ocean and the overpopulation of the world. Too bad no one dares to talk about human overpopulation as a cause of so many of the world's woes. Everyone is hung up on treating the symptoms.

Today is blustery, with heavy seas, wind and rain. I am content to stay in, because after work yesterday I trekked out to Tolstoi Point, where I had seen mossberries. I managed to pick enough to spread over vanilla ice cream for dessert. Wonderful! They are much more sweet and juicy than the ones around Anchorage.

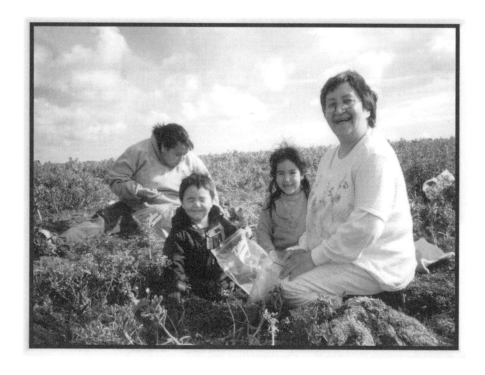

PAULINE RUKOVISHNIKOFF *(right), picking blueberries at St. Paul with daughter* FAITH *(left) and grandchildren* "BIG BOY" RAFAEL III *and* MARIA QUADELUPE.

St. Paul

Nov 17, 2009—Tuesday.

I AM HOUSED IN MY OLD ROOM AT THE new quarters and was just getting off work when who should walk in but Grace from St. George, here for a conference. We talked while fixing dinner (split pea soup for her and caribou meatloaf, baked potato and squash for me). Good to get follow-up on some of my patients. I asked about the girl with the enormous plantar wart. Her mother was treating it with wart-off of some kind, and I had told her it would take forever and probably not work for such a large and deep wart. She was going to Anchorage anyway so went to the family practice clinic there and they sent her to dermatology. Dermatology told them that family practice should have taken care of her and sent them back. The mother gave up and just took her home. Poor kid. I will see if this clinic can't lend them some equipment to do the job.

Busy here. Josh, the PA I hadn't met before, is excellent and very pleasant to work with. He is taking call all week until I can get my feet on the ground with all the new equipment. He also monitors the radios at night so when I'm on call he will be right over if he hears something serious. What a load that removes.

11-21-09

SATURDAY—I AM on call 24/7 until I leave, which may be next Friday, the day after Thanksgiving. Quiet so far today, and dear Pauline has promised to back me up if something serious comes in and I can't find the equipment I need. She invited me over for her famous fish pie—fantastic halibut plus a very good carrot raisin salad. There were two tables of relatives and me, with lots of talk and kids running around and the parakeet talking in the cage.

Beautiful weather earlier, with sun and no wind, but I had too much to do to even try walking out to the point beyond East Landing. It is barren of seals anyway. Now it is typical Pribilof weather, with gale winds blowing snow. No plane for three days. I needed crampons to get to the store for milk.

I had a good laugh yesterday. It was a little slower than usual because of the blizzard (no one wants to leave home), but from 1:30 to 2:30 the seniors exercise to a video in the waiting room. I decided I had better go. I entertained the others, who laughed along with me at my ineptitude. I am so pleased to see so much new exercise equipment, and all of it being used. They even have a TV in the corner up high so you can watch it while you work out. Very fancy.

A patient told me yesterday afternoon that they were having a movie, *People of the Seal*, which had won awards at several film festivals. I was so glad I went. The videos of the islands and the beaches with the tall grasses moved me to tears. I hate to think of retiring and not coming out here anymore. They must have had the Coast Guard helicopter for some of the scenes. It will be showing at the Bear Tooth Theater in Anchorage the week I get back. I will corner friends and family and go again.

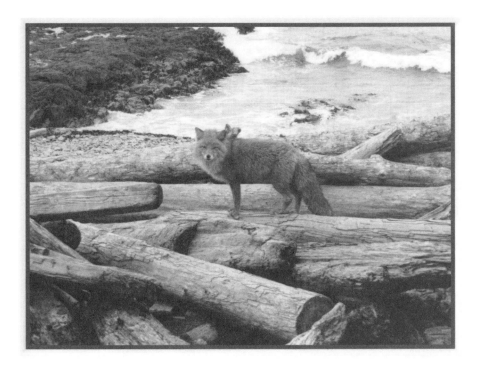

Amulet

I will chip the secrets of this day
from the stone cliffs soaring
above the restless sea.
Steal their half-heard whispers
and hold them deep within
next to the gull's cry,
the curve of the fox's tail,
the unstoppered attar
of salt—
to savor in the emptiness
of no return

Epilog

. .

O N MY 81ST BIRTHDAY, IN 2010, I retired from my work with the Aleutian/Pribilof Islands Association. As I reflect on the long and varied path that led to "the stone cliffs and the restless sea," I feel as if I am back in my darkroom on the farm in Lynden—the storage room on the landing next to my bedroom—developing rolls of film. When film is developed it is blank until the image gradually appears. Each image in turn shows what was hidden within but never what the next frame will be. I see again the uncertainty of what the future will bring that surrounded me the first year and a half of college, remembering how it dissolved when I decided to be a doctor.

Already I know that it isn't just the islands I will miss, but the people.

Clearly etched in the frame of my memory are those I have met in the past 20 years. Irene McGlashan, with her warm, open heart, going with me to visit a dying patient. Millie Prokopeuff, who always knew how to get things done. When circumstances were difficult for me, she calmly took the pressure off.

Dave Davelos, and the day we had five dislocated shoulders in a row. Mayor of Atka George Dirks, with his gentle, warm wisdom. Pauline Rukovishnikoff, who made me feel part of the family. Scott and Agrafina Kerr, ever helpful as well as generous with Whirlwind. Val and Pauline Dushkin, kind storehouses of Aleut culture. Adoptive Alaskans Abi and Marlaine and Cora, dear friends, along with

Cora's husband, Milt. Bone Lekanof. Peat Galaktionoff. The patients, the village health aides, the PA's and NP's and FNP's. Many are listed in the Index. Some I knew only by first name; some names I never knew.

Now I begin a new phase of my life—slower paced, with time for reflection. A frame, undeveloped, but like earlier images sure to be satisfying in its own way.

Resources

BOOKS:

The Alaska Medevac Manual: Guidelines for Medevac Escort, Karyn M.
Patno, M.D., and Becky Lundqvist, R.N. Alaska Dept. of Health
and Social Services, Division of Public Health, fifth printing.
(Note: The terms medevac and medivac are both accepted usage.)

Aleuts: Survivors of the Bering Land Bridge, William S. Laughlin.
Holt, Rinehart & Winston, 1980.

Moments Rightly Placed: An Aleutian Memoir, Raymond L. Hudson.
Epicenter Press, second printing, 2008.

*A New and Untried Course: Woman's Medical College and Medical College
of Pennsylvania, 1850-1998*, Steven J. Peitzman, M.D. Rutgers
University Press, 2000.

Umnak: The People Remember, Tyler M. Schlung and students
of Nikolski School. Hardscratch Press, 2003.

FILMS:

Aleut Evacuation: The Untold War Story. Produced by Michael and
Mary Jo Thill, Gaff Rigged Productions, and Dimitri Philemonof,
Aleutian/Pribilof Islands Association, Inc., 1992 (VHS).

People of the Seal: Pribilof Islands, Alaska, by Kate Raisz. Produced by
John A. Lindsay; narrated by Aquilina Lestenkof. NOAA Ocean
Media Center and 42°N Films, 2008 (DVD).

ARTICLES:

"Life on a Sheep Ranch in the Aleutians," by Len Dalton.
Melrose Mirror, Melrose, Idaho, July 2, 1999.
(On the Internet, search for "sheep ranch in the Aleutians"
to read the article online.)

Index of Names

Boldface *page numbers indicate photographs.*

A Small Glossary of Medical Terms

Anaphylaxis: a severe reaction to an allergen; common causes are drug or food allergies, or insect bites or stings. Anaphylaxis is life-threatening and can occur at any time.

Beta blocker: a class of drug used for treating abnormal heart rhythms, angina, high blood pressure, migraine, and other conditions.

Bolus: a dose of a substance (drug or medication) given intravenously.

Bundle branch block: a delay or blockage on the pathway that sends electrical impulses to the left or right side of the heart.

Crab asthma: an allergic, potentially life-threatening sensitivity to crab meat, shells, or even the steam from cooking.

Edema (four plus): swelling from an excessive accumulation of fluid in the tissues. The higher the number, the greater the swelling.

Endometriosis: a condition in which the tissue that normally lines the uterus grows somewhere else—commonly around the ovaries, behind the uterus or on the bowels or bladder; can cause pain, infertility, and very heavy periods.

Fascia: the sheath of fibrous tissue that envelops the body (beneath the skin).

Fecolith: a rounded pellet of feces.

Glucagon: a hormone produced by cells in the pancreas; helps control blood sugar levels. A glucagon test measures the amount of glucagon in the blood.

Gravida three: a woman in her third pregnancy.

Mucosa: the moist tissues that line body cavities, including the respiratory and gastrointestinal tracts.

NP (FNP): nurse practitioner (family nurse practitioner).

O_2 sats: oxygen saturation, referring to the level of oxygen carried by red blood cells through the arteries and delivered to internal organs. As red blood cells travel through the lungs, they are saturated with oxygen; a low saturation level could indicate a respiratory illness or other medical condition.

Orthopnea: shortness of breath.

PA (PA-C): physician's assistant (certified).

Periostium: the heavy membrane that covers the surface of bones.

Pleural effusion: a buildup of fluid between the layers of tissue that line the lungs and chest cavity.

Septic shock: a potentially lethal drop in blood pressure caused by the presence of bacteria in the blood.

Stertorous: a heavy "snoring" sound (as in a heart murmur).

Tachycardia: excessively rapid heartbeat.

Vagotomy: surgical procedure to control a duodenal ulcer.

Other books from Hardscratch Press

The Alaska 67: A Guide to Alaska's Best History Books, compiled by
the Alaska Historical Society. ISBN: 978-9-9678989-9-5.

Alaska Journey 1919–1934: An adventurous young Norwegian's coming-of-age, by Ralph Soberg (three earlier books in one volume: *Captain Hardscratch & Others, Survival on Montague Island, Confessions of an Alaska Bootlegger*). ISBN: 0-9625429-6-2.

Any Tonnage, Any Ocean: Conversations with a resolute Alaskan
(Capt. Walter Jackinsky Jr. of Ninilchik, 34-year veteran of the
Alaska Marine Highway System), compiled by Jacquelin Benson Pels.
ISBN: 0-9678989-5-1.

*Bridging Alaska / From the Big Delta to the Kenai: A personal account of
30 years of pioneer bridge and road construction throughout
the 49th state,* by Ralph Soberg. ISBN: 0-9625429-2-X.

The Dragline Kid: A gold miner's daughter from Hope, Alaska . . . ,
by Lisa Augustine. ISBN: 0-9678989-3-5. [Awaiting second printing.]

Family After All: Alaska's Jesse Lee Home (Vol. I, *Unalaska, 1889–1925,*
by Raymond L. Hudson, ISBN: 978-0-9789979-0-8; Vol. II, *Seward,
1925–1965,* compiled by Jacquelin B. Pels, ISBN: 978-0-9789979-1-5).

Gilbert Said: An oldtimer's tales of the Haida-Tlingit waterways of Alaska,
by Marian L. Swain. ISBN: 0-9625429-4-6.

*Homesteaders in the Headlights: One family's journey from a Depression-
era New Jersey farm to a new life in Wasilla, Alaska,*
by George Harbeson Jr. ISBN: 978-0-9789979-8-4.

Kachemak Bay Years: An Alaska homesteader's memoir, by Elsa Pedersen.
ISBN: 0-9678989-1-9.

*Miner, Preacher, Doctor, Teacher: Stories of an odyssey from Ann Arbor,
Mich., to Ketchikan, Alaska, to a pioneering medical career in
Oakland, Calif.,* compiled by Lee Sims. ISBN: 0-9625429-9-7.

Umnak: The People Remember, compiled by Tyler M. Schlung and students
of Nikolski School, Umnak Island, Alaska. ISBN: 0-9678989-4-3.

Unga Island Girl [Ruth's Book], by J.R.B. Pels. ISBN: 0-9625429-7-0.
[Out of print.]

CALIFORNIA:

All the Best: The Life of Victor M. Carter, by Dr. Fanya Carter.
ISBN: 978-0-9678989-8-8.

*Autumn Loneliness: The Letters of Kiyoshi & Kiyoko Tokutomi,
July–December 1967,* translated by Tei Matsushita Scott and
Patricia J. Machmiller, ISBN: 978-0-9789979-4-6.

Historic Livermore, California, A–Z, by Anne Marshall Homan.
ISBN: 978-0-9789979-8-9.

The Life Story of Henry Ramsey Jr., by Judge Henry Ramsey Jr. of Rocky
Mount, N.C., and Berkeley, Calif. ISBN: 978-0-9789979-3-9.

*The Morning Side of Mount Diablo: An illustrated account of the San
Francisco Bay Area's historic Morgan Territory Road,*
by Anne Marshall Homan. ISBN: 0-9678989-2-7.

Vasco's Livermore, 1910: Portraits from the Hub Saloon,
by Anne Marshall Homan and Richard W. Finn.
ISBN: 978-9789979-7-7.

NEW ENGLAND:

Circuses & Sailing Ships: Recollections of a Runaway New England Boy,
by Nelson F. Getchell. ISBN: 0-9678989-0-0.

*Fin, Fur & Fiber: The life and [fishing] times of a New England
textile man,* by Nelson F. Getchell. ISBN: 978-0-9678989-6-4.

*MCML / Mary Cole Mason Lord, 1887–1988: A sampler of stories
from a turn-of-the-century girlhood in Marblehead, Mass.,*
by Martha Mason Lord Getchell. ISBN: 0-9625429-5-4.

FOR CHILDREN (IN SPANISH AND ENGLISH):

*Cuando llegabas, nieto mío / La valiente hermana mayor (When you were
on your way, grandson / The brave big sister),* by J.R.B. Pels.
ISBN: 0-9625429-8-9. [Out of print.]

About the Author

IN A LETTER DATED JULY 7, 1945, 16-year-old Nancy Elliott wrote to a former teacher: "... from now on my money goes into flying lessons. Last Saturday Don, Art, Kenny and I went to the Lakeside Air Service for a 15-minute instruction. You couldn't keep me on the ground with anything but lack of money now. We actually got to take over the controls and mess around. It takes off at 50 mph, climbs at 60 and cruises at 90. We went up to 1,000 feet and then I took over. I banked and looked down. Believe it or not I could see all the rest of the kids down below. That 15 minutes was the shortest 15 minutes in my life. I hope I make it to solo. ... "

Required for the flight was the purchase of a $100 war bond. The future pilot picked strawberries through the summer and worked nights in a cannery to earn the $75 cost of the bond. Twenty years later, after studying for her M.D. at the pioneering and prestigious Woman's Medical College of Pennsylvania, she did indeed "make it to solo," and beyond—between pregnancies the mother of four had earned her land and sea rating.

· ·

IN 1988, DR. NANCY ELLIOTT SYDNAM left a thriving family practice in Anchorage to travel and tend to what Ray Hudson in the Foreword calls "one of the most diverse and remote regions of Alaska." This book, a collection of journal entries, letters, poems and commentary, follows her on her perilous rounds.

About the 1945 description of that first flight, she wrote in 2012: "Sally Siemons (her real first name was Alice) was my sixth-grade teacher who moved to Seattle. I think I wanted to write but thought the only way to write was to send letters; I had always admired her

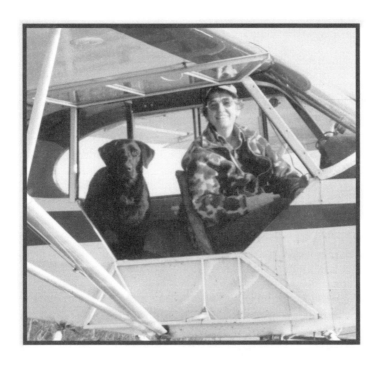

so started to write to her. Before she died she sent me all the letters I had written. I was amazed that she had kept them." Readers of *Sideways Rain* will be grateful to teacher Siemons for tacitly encouraging the fledgling writer.

("She was an excellent teacher," Nancy wrote. "I especially admired her for telling off one of the boys in the class when he announced that he thought she was not worth knowing and that he thoroughly despised her. She just looked him right in the eye and said, 'The feeling is entirely mutual.' Poor kid didn't know what mutual meant.")

Jackie Pels
Hardscratch Press
November 2012

SIDEWAYS RAIN
*20 years of medicine, music, and good-luck landings
in the Aleutian and Pribilof Islands of Alaska*

Project coordinator and editor: JACKIE PELS

Book design and production: DAVID R. JOHNSON

Typography and composition: DICKIE MAGIDOFF

Proofreading and photo scans: LEAH H. PELS

CIP data by ROSE SCHREIER WELTON, M.L.S.

Thanks to Daryl Moistner for the use of his Aleutians photographs on the cover and within, and to Clare Lattimore,
Pauline Rukovishnikoff, Millie Prokopeuff, Abi Woodbridge,
Peat Galaktionoff, Shelly and Ray Hudson, and Aquilina Lestenkof
for help with names of people and places in the narrative.
The passage from the film *People of the Seal* on page 80
is quoted with Aquilina's permission.

Printed and bound at McNAUGHTON & GUNN,
Saline, Michigan

Alkaline pH paper (Natural Offset)

HARDSCRATCH PRESS
658 Francisco Court
Walnut Creek, CA 94598-2213

925/935-3422

[HARDSCRATCH]
www.hardscratchpress.com